Pulmonary Physiology for Pre-Clinical Students

Instructor Resources

How to Adopt This Book

This is an open textbook. That means that this book is freely available and you are welcome to use, adapt, and share this book with attribution according to the Creative Commons NonCommercial ShareAlike 4.0 (CC BY-NC-SA 4.0) license https://creativecommons.org/licenses/by-nc-sa/4.0. (Many, but not all images, illustrations, etc in this book are licensed under CC BY 4.0.)

Instructors reviewing, adopting, or adapting this textbook are encouraged to register at https://bit.ly/interest-preclinical. This assists the Open Education Initiative at Virginia Tech in assessing the impact of the book and allows us to more easily alert instructors of additional resources, features and opportunities.

Finding Additional Resources for Your Course

The main landing page for the book is https://pressbooks.lib.vt.edu/pulmonaryphysiology.

This page includes:

- Links to multiple electronic versions of the textbook (PDF, ePub, HTML)
- Links to the instructor resource-sharing portal
- Link to errata document (report errors at https://bit.ly/feedback-preclinical)
- Links to other books within this series

Sharing Resources You've Created

Have you created any supplementary materials for use with Cardiovascular Pathophysiology for Pre-Clinical Students such as presentation slides, activities, test items, or a question bank? If so, please consider sharing your materials related to this open textbook. Please tell us about resources you wish to share by using this form: https://bit.ly/interest-preclinical or by directly sharing resources under an open license to the public-facing instructor sharing portal https://www.oercommons.org/groups/pre-clinical-resources/10133.

Customizing This Book

The Creative Commons Attribution NonCommercial-ShareAlike 4.0 license https://creativecommons.org/licenses/by-nc-sa/4.0/legalcode on this book allows customization and redistribution which is NonCommercial, that is "not primarily intended for or directed towards commercial advantage or monetary compensation."

Best practices for attribution are provided at https://wiki.creativecommons.org/wiki/ Best_practices_for_attribution.

This book is hosted in PDF and ePub in VTechWorks http://hdl.handle.net/10919/105410 in HTML in Pressbooks https://pressbooks.lib.vt.edu/pulmonaryphysiology and via the LibreTexts platform https://med.libretexts.org/@go/page/34378. Pressbooks and LibreTexts platforms both offer customization/remixing.

Pulmonary Physiology for Pre-Clinical Students

ANDREW BINKS

PDF AND EPUB FREE ONLINE AT: HTTPS://DOI.ORG/10.21061/PULMONARYPHYSIOLOGY

VTC | Virginia Tech Carilion School of Medicine

VIRGINIA TECH PUBLISHING

VIRGINIA TECH CARILION SCHOOL OF MEDICINE IN ASSOCIATION WITH VIRGINIA TECH PUBLISHING
BLACKSBURG, VA

Suggested citation: Binks, Andrew (2022). *Pulmonary Physiology for Pre-Clinical Students*. Roanoke: Virginia Tech Carilion School of Medicine. https://doi.org/10.21061/pulmonaryphysiology. Licensed with CC BY-NC-SA 4.0 https://creativecommons.org/licenses/by-nc-sa/4.0.

Publisher: This work is published by the Virginia Tech Carilion School of Medicine in association with Virginia Tech Publishing, a division of the University Libraries at Virginia Tech.

Virginia Tech Carilion School of Medicine 2 Riverside Circle Roanoke, VA 24016 USA

Virginia Tech Publishing University Libraries at Virginia Tech 560 Drillfield Drive Blacksburg, VA 24061 USA https://publishing.vt.edu publishing@vt.edu

This work is also distributed by LibreTexts, Davis, CA USA info@libretexts.org. Note: The LibreTexts version of this work at https://med.libretexts.org/@go/page/34378 may differ from this version.

Peer review: This book has undergone single-blind peer review by two external reviewers.

Accessibility statement: Virginia Tech Publishing is committed to making its publications accessible in accordance with the Americans with Disabilities Act of 1990. The Pressbooks (HTML) and ePub versions of this text are tagged structurally and include alternative text, which allows for machine readability.

Publication cataloging information:
Binks, Andrew, author
Pulmonary Physiology for Pre-Clinical Students / Andrew Binks
Pages cm
ISBN 978-1-957213-12-5 (PDF)
ISBN 978-1-957213-14-9 (ePub)
ISBN 978-1-957213-15-6 (Pressbooks) https://pressbooks.lib.vt.edu/pulmonaryphysiology
ISBN 978-1-957213-13-2 (Print)
URI (Universal Resource Identifier): http://hdl.handle.net/10919/105410
DOI https://doi.org/10.21061/pulmonaryphysiology

1. Lungs -- Physiology -- Textbooks
2. Respiration -- Textbooks
   Title QP107 .B56 2022

Cover art: Lungs by iconmu via the Noun Project. CC BY 3.0.
Illustration and cover design: Kindred Grey

Contents

Introduction

Pulmonary disease is one of the prevalent clinical issues that graduating health care professionals will address. The purpose of this book is to provide an understanding of the basic concepts of common diseases of the pulmonary system in preparation for professional exams and the clinic.

Pulmonary Physiology for Pre-Clinical Students, is an undergraduate medical-level resource for foundational knowledge of common pulmonary diseases, disorders and pathologies. This text is designed for a course pre-clinical undergraduate medical curriculum and it is aligned to USMLE(r) (United States Medical Licensing Examination) content guidelines. The text is meant to provide the essential information from these content areas in a concise format that would allow learner preparation to engage in an active classroom. Clinical correlates and additional application of content is intended to be provided in the classroom experience. This resource should be assistive to the learner later in medical school and for exam preparation given the material is presented in a succinct manner, with a focus on high-yield concepts.

Pulmonary Physiology for Pre-Clinical Students is intended to address both necessary content and align with the preclerkship curricular needs. The utility of a flexible text can positively impact the learning environment and increase student engagement and performance. This text is made to be adaptable by using pieces and parts to suit students and inspire the addition of elements to this living resource.

Features of this Book

- Detailed learning objectives are provided at the beginning of each subsection
- High resolution, color contrasting figures illustrate concepts, relationships, and processes throughout
- Summary tables display detailed information
- Accessibility features including structured heads and alternative-text provide access for readers accessing the work via a screen-reader

This resource was designed to fill a gap in undergraduate medical education (UME) and support preclerkship education in the content areas of basic science for medical education. Unlike traditional textbooks, the organization of this resource is driven by curricular structure, rather than subject area. As the format and design of UME differs across many programs, this resource is purposefully brief and flexible, allowing for rapid adaptation across programs. The resource is organized into small chapters that can be used to support student preparation in any arrangement. The sections are not intended to be all-inclusive, but rather primers for applied content delivery. In our curriculum, these topic areas are interwoven into problem-based and case based learning modalities. The cases and clinical correlates change regularly and having the flexibility of these short resources that can be applied to many scenarios across the pre-clinical years of our curriculum is beneficial.

Over the past twenty years, medical education has undergone a rapid curricular restructuring. This is in part due to recommendations of the Flexner report[1], coupled with the changes observed in millennial[2] and iGen learners. To accommodate the integration of additional core competencies, the majority of medical programs have moved away from discipline-based delivery and currently use some form of integrated curricular format.[3] This allows material to be presented in a more clinically realistic and pertinent format without the constraints of artificial discipline silos. This movement has had positive impacts on programmatic outcomes and student performance, but it has presented some challenges for curricular design, student engagement and educational resources.

Although contemporary medical curricula have moved to a cohesive, integrated format, the required textbooks for undergraduate medical education remain traditional and discipline-based. Use of small, independent chapters allows content to be delivered in a variety of curricular settings and support content integration and alignment.

A high volume of content, some of it lacking alignment with class sessions coupled with restrictions on student contact time imposed by accrediting bodies, means that faculty across the country are having to rethink preparation materials to facilitate efficient, focused learning experiences. This resource It is intended to provide learners with a high-level view of relevant topical areas that will be further elaborated on within the classroom setting. Unlike other traditional textbooks, it is not intended to include all content a learner would need about the relevant subject area but to function as a stepping stone towards mastery of the content.

As programs embrace the philosophy of student-directed learning embedded in adult learning theory, more simplified readily available resources will be essential to support this fast-paced learning of health professional educational programs. While there are many factors that can contribute to a student's lack of preparation, lengthy textbook resources for a single integrated classroom session have a significant negative impact. So while an integrated curricular model enhances many aspects of learning, it makes using traditional textbooks cumbersome and disjointed for students. This resource hopes to address this concern.

Finally, there is a wealth of "medical" content freely accessible online, and students can find themselves spending a significant amount of time trying to identify alternative resources that may—or may not—be appropriate. Faculty taking ownership to identify and adapt realistic materials for each session reduces the concern that students are finding misinformation through internet sources, and this project allows faculty to create a resource that harnesses the best attributes of many different formats into a product that best supports the learning environment. Otherwise, external online resources are also likely to contain extraneous content that is not aligned with the classroom learning objectives (akin to subject-based textbook chapters), so it can also reduce the perceived worth of preparation. If the integrated resource is generated correctly, concisely and accurately by the faculty, the students will gain trust, rely on the vetted resources and prepare for the active classroom.

References

1. Cooke M, Irby DM, Ph D, et al. American Medical Education 100 Years after the Flexner Report. 2006: 1339-1344.
2. Roberts DH, Newman LR, Schwartzstein RM. Twelve tips for facilitating Millennials' learning. Medical Teacher. 2012; 34: 274-278.
3. VanTassel-Baska J, Wood S. The integrated curriculum model (ICM). Learning and Individual Differences. 2010; 20(4): 345-357.

About the Author

Dr. Andrew Binks is a cardiopulmonary physiologist who gained his BSc (Hons) in Physiological Sciences at the University of Newcastle upon Tyne, then a MSc in Human and Applied Physiology from King's College, London. He returned to Newcastle to do his PhD and study the underlying physiological mechanisms of dyspnea, the cardinal symptom of cardiopulmonary disease. He continued investigating dyspnea at Harvard School of Public Health as a postdoctoral fellow and then as a research scientist. After seven years at Harvard, Andrew took his first faculty position at the University of New England where he taught cardiovascular and pulmonary physiology to health profession and medical students. He continued to teach medical students their heart and lung physiology after moving to the University of South Carolina's Medical School in Greenville where he also directed the school's heart and lung pathophysiology courses. Andrew currently teaches heart and lung physiology and pathophysiology at Virginia Tech Carilion School of Medicine, directs the heart and lung pathophysiology course and has also served as the departmental director of faculty development.

In his two decades of teaching medical physiology, Andrew has regularly drawn upon his dyspnea research experience to generate an active, clinically focused approach to medical education. This book is part of that approach and supports students preparing for class with the basic information with the intention to apply and contextualize that information in a guided case-based classroom experience.

Andrew has published numerous peer-reviewed research papers and book chapters about dyspnea and about contemporary medical education. He has also given keynote presentations, faculty workshops and international webinars to promote effective medical education for the modern adult learner.

Acknowledgments

Funding and In-Kind Support
Publication of this work is made possible in part through the support of VIVA (Virtual Library of Virginia), LibreTexts, the Open Education Initiative of the University Libraries at Virginia Tech, and Virginia Tech Publishing.

Peer Reviewers
Alex Atwood, Medical Resident
Michael North, Medical Resident

Editorial Team
Managing Editor: Anita Walz
Graphic Design and Editorial Assistance: Kindred Grey
Alternative Text: Andrew Binks

Special Thanks
Delmar Larson, Founder, LibreTexts
Christa Miller, Accessible Technologies, Virginia Tech

About the Author

1. Fundamentals

Learning objectives

- Relate the anatomy of the airways, airspaces and cellular structure of the lungs to lung function.

The Components of Lung Function

The primary function of the pulmonary system is to maintain arterial blood gas homeostasis by gaining oxygen from the atmosphere and expelling carbon dioxide from the venous blood. Although initially appearing simple, this process is a summation of distinct components that are important to understand if one is to understand the mechanisms and management of pulmonary diseases. Each of these components are shown in the schematic of figure 1.1 and are addressed chapter by chapter in this book.

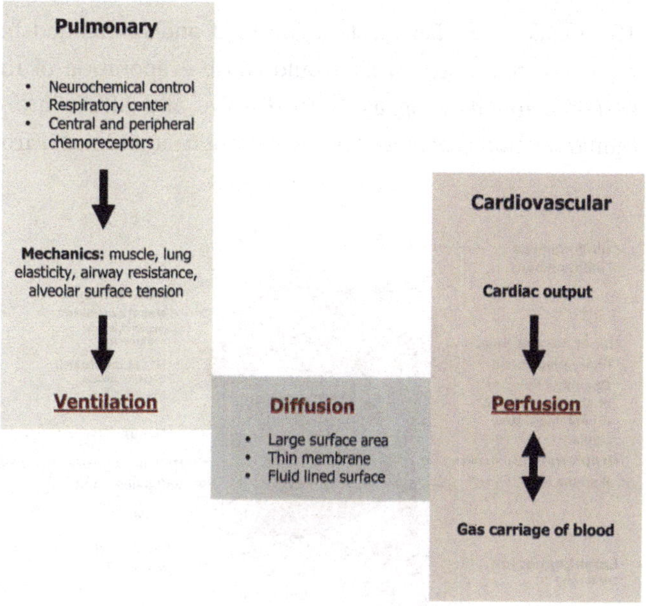

Figure 1.1: Components of gas exchange.

We will see how blood gases are monitored and maintained through neurochemical control of lung expansion and relaxation to achieve the appropriate level of alveolar ventilation. Factors that affect the degree of gas exchange between the lung and blood will be discussed, along with the coordination of ventilation and perfusion of the lung. Finally, we will see how oxygen and carbon dioxide are transported in the bloodstream to and from tissue and the mechanisms that ensure appropriate delivery and a stable blood gas environment. Before we begin, however, we will look at the functional anatomy of the lung and how the lung is well designed to perform its primary role and defend itself from the external environment.

Defense of the Lung

As the only internal organ exposed to the external environment, the lung needs special protection from particles or pathogens that could be transported down the airways with inhaled air. The first line of defense is the nasal cavity, which is lined with a ciliated epithelial, dispersed within which are goblet cells producing mucus (figure 1.2). This mucus forms a sticky layer on top of the epithelial surface and traps inhaled particles, bacteria, or other potential pathogens. The mucus is then moved by the cilia back toward the pharynx where it can be coughed or spat out.

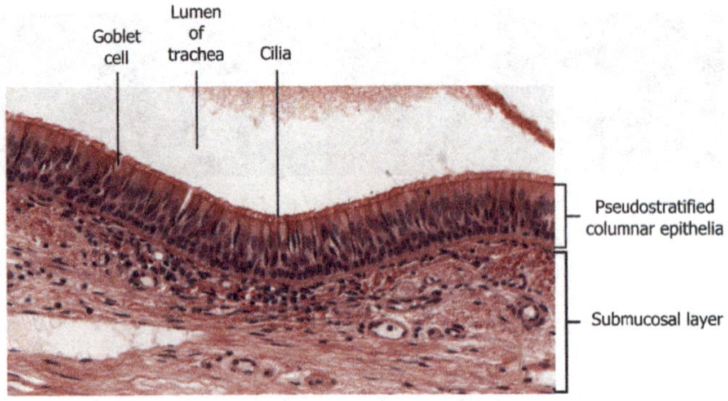

Figure 1.2: The mucociliary escalator of the airway. The cilia on the apical surface of the pseudostratified epithelium push a layer of mucus (produced by the goblet cells) toward the mouth, carrying pathogens and particulates out of the airway.

The inhaled air also must be warmed and humidified before it reaches the gas exchange surfaces, otherwise the relatively cold and dry air would cause evaporation of the thin water layer lining the gas exchange surfaces that is essential for allowing gases to dissolve and diffuse into or out of the pulmonary bloodstream. This warming and humidification is achieved by transfer of heat and water from blood in the highly vascularized nasal cavity (figure 1.3).

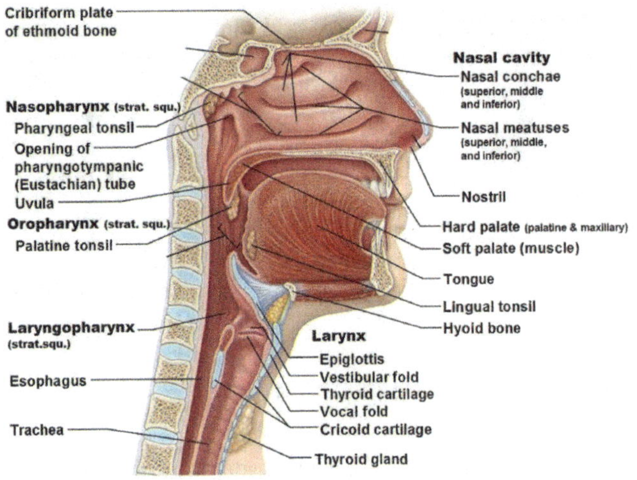

Figure 1.3: Air conditioning. The highly vascularized nasal cavity helps warm and humidify inhaled air before it proceeds toward the lower airways.

The second line of defense (which becomes more important when breathing through the mouth) is the lining of the trachea. Again, this is covered with a ciliated epithelium with mucus-producing goblet cells (figure 1.2). As in the nasal cavity, particles and potential pathogens are trapped in the mucus layer and cilia move the mucus up toward the mouth for expulsion. The trachea and larynx also contain sensory nerve endings (rapidly adapting receptors, nicknamed "irritant receptors") that respond to the arrival of particles on the epithelial surface and initiate the cough reflex and propel the offending particles out of the airway (see more in chapter 17).

The Bronchial Tree

The airways, or bronchial tree (figure 1.4), consist of a series of branching tubes that become narrower and shorter but more numerous as they descend into the lung.

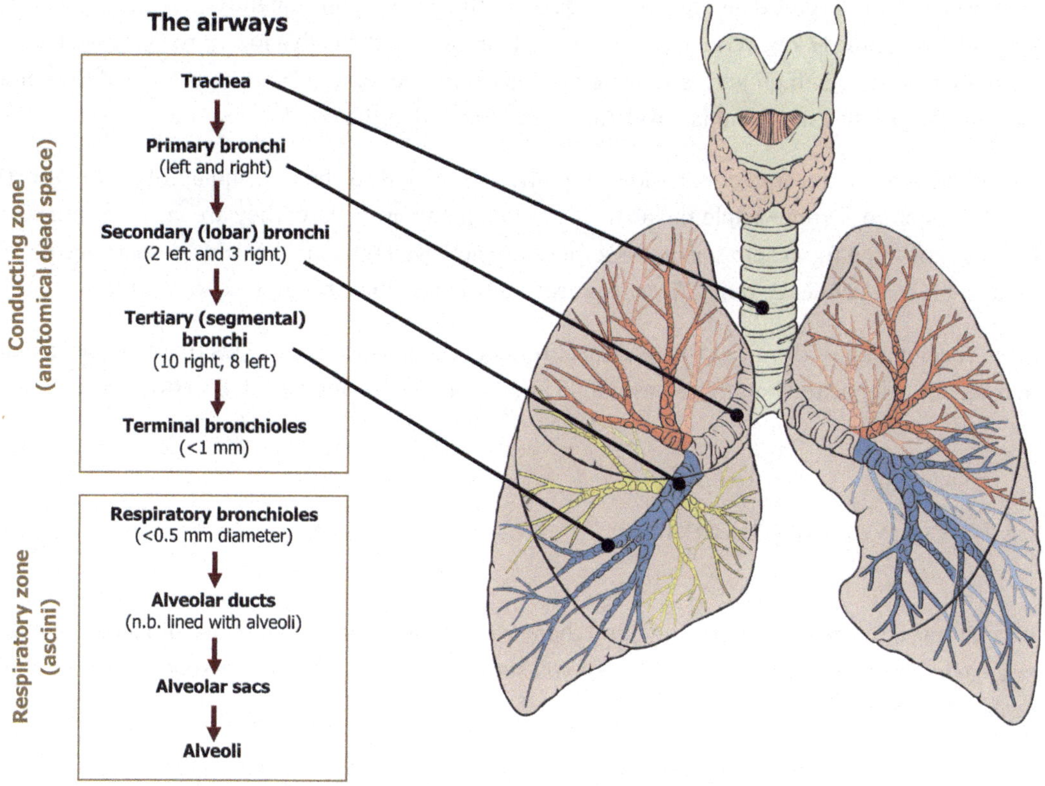

Figure 1.4: The bronchial tree. The major airways of the conducting zone (anatomical dead space) are labeled.

The trachea bifurcates into the primary bronchi, left and right, transporting air into the left and right lungs, respectively. The primary bronchi consequently divide into lobar (or secondary) bronchi, the number of which correspond to the number of lobes in each lung. The lobar bronchi then divide into segmental (or tertiary) bronchi to supply the segments of each lobe. This bifurcation process continues to the terminal bronchioles. This initial section of the bronchial tree is referred to as the *conducting zone* as its role is to transfer air to the gas exchange surfaces (figure 1.4). As no gas exchange takes place here, these airways constitute the *anatomical dead space* and have a volume of approximately 150 mL.

Each terminal bronchiole then divides into numerous respiratory bronchioles, the walls of which may contain some alveoli and are therefore capable of some gas exchange; this is the transition to the *respiratory zone* of the lung and the onset of gas exchange (figure 1.4). The respiratory zone becomes firmly established when terminal bronchioles divide into alveolar ducts that are fundamentally tubes lined with alveoli. These alveolar ducts then terminate in alveolar sacs. The portion of lung distal to each terminal bronchiole forms an anatomical unit called the acinus. Although only a few millimeters long, collectively these acini make up the respiratory zone and form the vast majority of the lung's volume.

Flow in the Airways

Airflow down the bronchial tree is caused by the generation of a pressure differential when lung volume is expanded by contraction of the respiratory muscles (more on this in chapter 2). Inspired air first enters the airways of the conducting zone, which while having the largest diameter airways also has the fewest; consequently the total cross-sectional area of the conducting zone is relatively low. With a large volume of air passing through a low cross-sectional area, the velocity of air in the conducting zone is high and is moving by "bulk flow" generated by the pressure differential (like water through a hose) until it reaches the terminal bronchioles and the end of the conducting zone.

When this air enters the respiratory zone, it slows rapidly. This is due to the enormous total cross-sectional area of the airways in the respiratory zone—while the airways are much narrower here, they are far more numerous. The final transfer of the gases through the respiratory zone is therefore achieved by diffusion; the rate of diffusion is so rapid and the distances so short that concentration differences are abolished within a second.

As an aside, this deceleration of the air at the terminal bronchioles means any particles that have been able to descend this deep are frequently deposited here. This has ramifications for disease and also delivery of inhaled medications.

Primary Objective: Gas Exchange

Gases that have diffused to the respiratory zone find themselves in an ideal environment for gas exchange. We will deal with gas exchange in more detail later (chapter 7), but you should appreciate that the essential components for efficient gas exchange are all present in the lung.

A large surface area is generated by the 500 million alveoli, and while each alveolus only has a diameter of 0.3 mm, collectively they produce a total gas exchange surface of 100 m^2—about the surface area of a tennis court.

The membranes that gases transfer across are very thin and pose little opposition. In brief, oxygen entering the alveolus only has to cross the squamous cell of the alveolus wall, a very thin basement membrane, and then the squamous cell of the capillary wall to get into the pulmonary circulation. The total distance can be as low as 0.2 micrometers. This degree of thinness also makes these membranes prone to damage.

As well as the alveolus receiving air (that is being ventilated), the other essential component for gas exchange is blood flow. This is provided by the pulmonary circulation and consists of all cardiac output coming from the right heart. The pulmonary circulation forms very dense networks of capillaries surrounding each alveolus, so much so that the alveoli can be imagined as being washed over with blood.

These characteristics make the lung a highly efficient exchange organ between the environment and the circulation, which is ideal for the transfer of O_2 into the bloodstream and, just as importantly, CO_2 out. It also allows some drugs to be delivered by inhalation, but also has the potential to allow noxious substances into the bloodstream. Likewise, changes in any of these characteristics of the lung in disease, such as loss of surface area in emphysema or membrane thickening in pulmonary fibrosis, can severely diminish gas exchange.

References, Resources, and Further Reading

Text

Levitsky, Michael G. “Chapter 1: Function and Structure of the Respiratory System.” In *Pulmonary Physiology*, 9th ed. New York: McGraw Hill Education, 2018.

West, John B. “Chapter 1: Structure and Function—How the Architecture of the Lung Subserves Its Function.” In *Respiratory Physiology: The Essentials*, 9th ed. Philadelphia: Wolters Kluwer Health/Lippincott Williams and Wilkins, 2012.

Widdicombe, John G., and Andrew S. Davis. “Chapter 1.” In *Respiratory Physiology*. Baltimore: University Park Press, 1983.

Figures

Figure 1.1: Components of gas exchange. Grey, Kindred. 2022. CC BY 4.0. https://archive.org/details/1.1_20220125/mode/1up

Figure 1.2: The mucociliary escalator. OpenStax College. 2013. CC BY 3.0. https://commons.wikimedia.org/wiki/File:2304_Pseudostratified_Epithelium.jpg

Figure 1.3: Air conditioning. Chukquemeka, Uchechukwu. 2018. “Free to be used and shared.” https://www.physio-pedia.com/File:Upper_respiratory_system_2.jpg#filelinks

Figure 1.4: The bronchial tree. Grey, Kindred. 2022. CC BY 4.0. Added Lung by Lynch, Patrick J. from WikimediaCommons. https://archive.org/details/1.5._20220125/mode/1up

2. Mechanics of the Lungs

Learning objectives

- Describe the changes in pleural and alveolar pressures and lung volume caused by contraction of respiratory muscles over the respiratory cycle.

Fundamentals of Gas Movement

This chapter describes the mechanisms by which air is moved into and out of the lung, or pulmonary mechanics.

Before we get into the details of how we breathe in, let me make sure we are all on the same page by going right back to basics, so bare with me or skip ahead if you are happy with pressure, volume, and flow.

To get air to move into the lungs we need to generate a pressure differential; that is the pressure inside the lungs must be lower than the pressure outside (i.e., atmospheric pressure), so that air moves down the pressure gradient into the lungs.

The low pressure inside the lungs is generated by increasing lung volume; bigger volume means fewer molecules in the same space, and therefore lower pressure (go back and revisit Boyle's law if needed).

The basis of inspiration is lowering lung pressure below atmospheric pressure, so that atmospheric pressure pushes air down the airways until pressure equilibrates. So the fundamental first step is, how do we increase lung volume?

To understand the mechanics of breathing we have to deal with two concepts: first how the action of the respiratory muscles increases thoracic volume, and second (and more complex) we need to understand the interaction of the lungs and the thoracic wall.

Let us deal with the respiratory muscles and expansion of the thorax first.

Changing Thoracic Volume

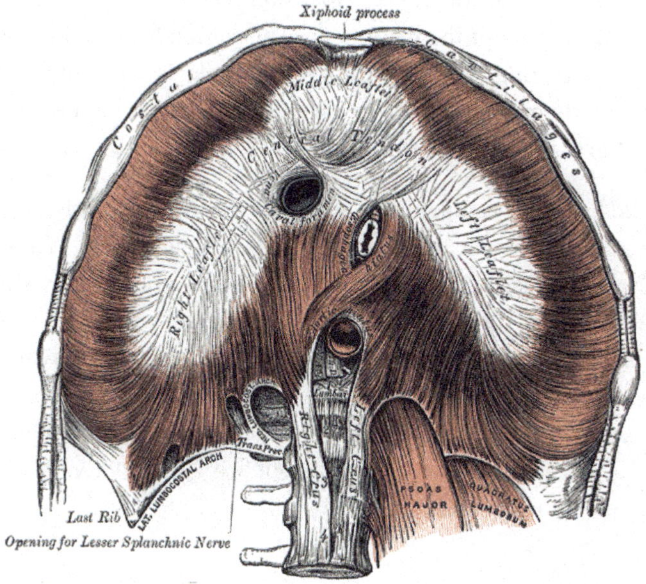

Figure 2.1: The diaphragm.

The muscle that generates the greatest change in thoracic volume (and thereby the greatest contribution to breathing) is the diaphragm (figure 2.1). Separating the thoracic and abdominal cavities, this sheetlike muscle forms a dome shape in the relaxed state that encroaches into the thorax. This sheet is formed of three sections, the anterior portion originating at the ribs and sternum, and the posterior portion originating on the vertebrae. These are connected by the central portion that is comprised of a tendon sheet.

It is worth a quick reminder that while controlling a visceral organ and performing a homeostatic function, the diaphragm and the other respiratory muscles are skeletal muscle and have the force-generation characteristics of such. As well as being under reflex control, it can also be controlled voluntarily (such as during speech).

Activation of the phrenic nerve stimulates the diaphragm and generates inspiration. Upon stimulation the contracting diaphragm flattens out, descending toward the abdomen. As it does so the thoracic volume increases, and consequently thoracic pressure falls. When thoracic pressure falls below atmospheric pressure, air moves down the generated pressure gradient and enters the lung. Note that this increase in thoracic volume comes at the expense of the abdominal volume, and abdominal contents can be compressed during inspiration. The diaphragm may descend as much as 10 cm, but a descent of 1 cm is sufficient to provide tidal breathing (figure 2.2).

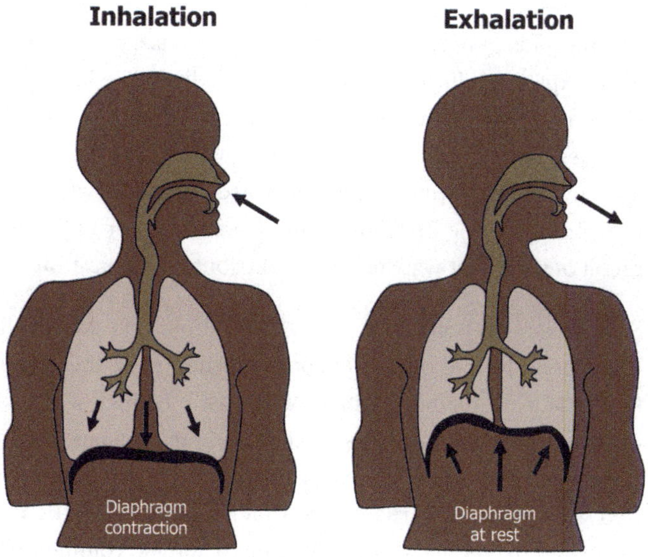

Figure 2.2: Diaphragm positional change.

When phrenic nerve activity stops, the diaphragm relaxes and returns to its resting dome-like position; this is aided by the recoil of the expanded lung and the decompression of the abdominal contents. The return to the resting position reduces thoracic volume and increases thoracic pressure above atmospheric pressure and air exits the lung down the reversed pressure gradient.

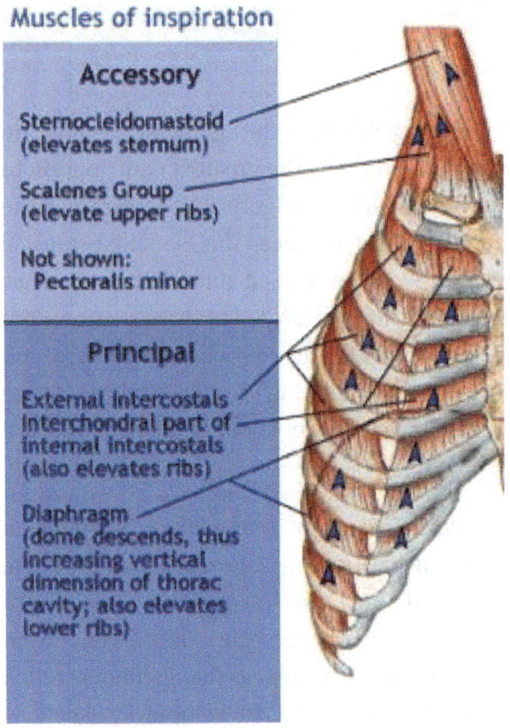

Figure 2.3: Inspiratory muscles of the rib cage.

During inspiration the thoracic volume is also increased by the action of the external intercostal muscles. Controlled by the intercostal nerve, contraction of the external intercostals causes the rib cage to rise upward and outward, resulting in an expansion of the thoracic volume in addition to the action of the diaphragm. This action is generated by the oblique positioning of the external intercostals between the ribs, and the sternum and upper ribs are stabilized by simultaneous activation of the scalenus muscles.

During periods of high ventilatory need (or drive) other muscles can contribute to expansion of the rib cage (figure 2.3). These "accessory" muscles assist the external intercostals and include the sternocleidomastoids, the scalenes, and the pectoralis minor. All of these groups allow for a greater thoracic expansion and thus a greater lung volume. Recognizing that a patient is using these muscles to breath is a useful clinical sign; use of these muscles during rest is highly indicative of a raised respiratory effort to cope with an underlying and probably significant problem.

Expiration is generally simpler. The elastic tissue of the lung has been expanded during inspiration, and a little like letting go of a stretch elastic band, the lungs recoil when the inspiratory muscles relax. This recoil reduces lung volume and increases lung pressure above atmospheric pressure and air exits the lung. Depending on the final lung volume achieved during inspiration, recoil of the chest wall may also contribute to expiration.

So during quiet resting breathing, expiration is passive, relying on the expenditure of the stored, potential energy in the elastic lung tissue. However, when ventilation needs to be increased, such as during exercise, this process is too slow, and this passive process needs some active help in order to increase the rate of breathing. Activation of the internal intercostal muscles draws the rib cage downward to reduce thoracic volume. Thoracic volume is further decreased by contraction of muscles surrounding the abdomen; these increase abdominal pressure and help push the diaphragm upward (figure 2.4).

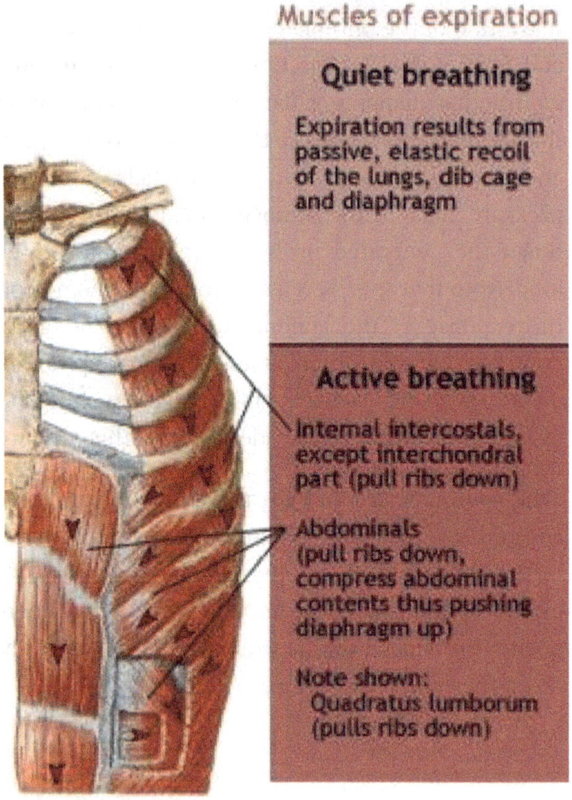

Figure 2.4: Expiratory muscles.

How the Lungs Move with the Chest Wall

Now having dealt with the expansion of the thoracic cage, we should look at the relationship between the thoracic wall and the lungs and how the lungs and the inside of the thorax are adhered to each other so when the thoracic wall moves the lungs follow.

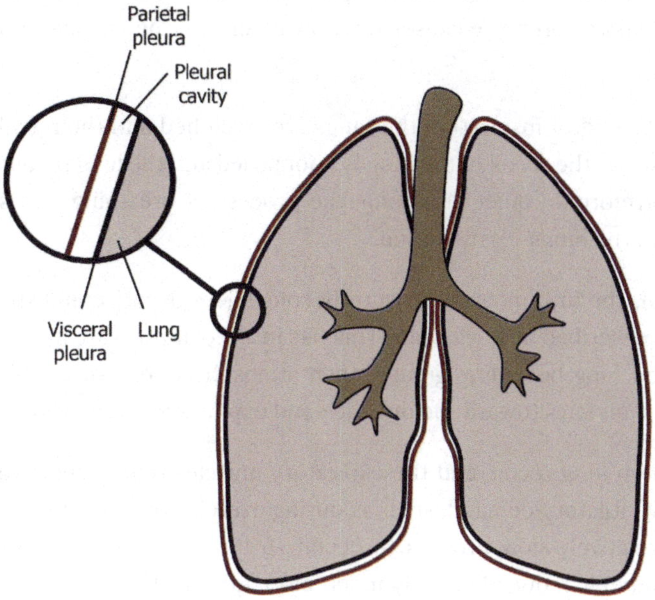

Figure 2.5: The pleural membranes and space.

The inside of the thoracic cavity is lined with a membrane, the parietal pleura. The outside of the lungs are lined with a membrane called the visceral pleura. The space between these membranes, the pleural cavity or pleural space, is filled with pleural fluid (figure 2.5). Normally there is only 5–10 mL of pleural fluid to cover all the lung's external surface. So the fluid layer and the intra-pleural space is extremely thin. When a thin layer of fluid is trapped between two surfaces it exerts surface tension and holds the two surfaces together; if you've ever been doing the washing up and trapped a layer of water between too dinner plates you'll have noticed its difficult to pry the plates apart. It is similar for the pleural membranes, and it is this surface tension that holds the outside of the lungs to the inside of the thorax. We will deal with surface tension in more detail in a later chapter.

We have mentioned the pressure inside the lungs, but now we have to think about the pressure inside the pleural space—called intra-pleural pressure. Even at normal, resting lung volumes the elastic tissue in the lungs is already somewhat stretched, so the lungs have a tendency to recoil, pulling inward. The chest wall, alternatively, has a tendency to spring outward. These opposing movements are prevented by the surface tension in the pleural space and cause a negative intrapleural pressure, that is below atmospheric pressure.

We should now consider what happens to intrapleural and airway pressures during the breathing cycle. First, let us look at the pressures and volumes before inspiration begins (figure 2.6). The intrapleural pressure is slightly negative (−5 cm H_2O) due to the recoil of the lung and outward spring of the chest wall. Before the breath starts lung volume is considered zero and flow is also zero (i.e., volume has not changed and there is no movement of air in the airways). Alveolar pressure, the pressure inside the lungs, is also zero, really meaning it is equal to atmospheric pressure.

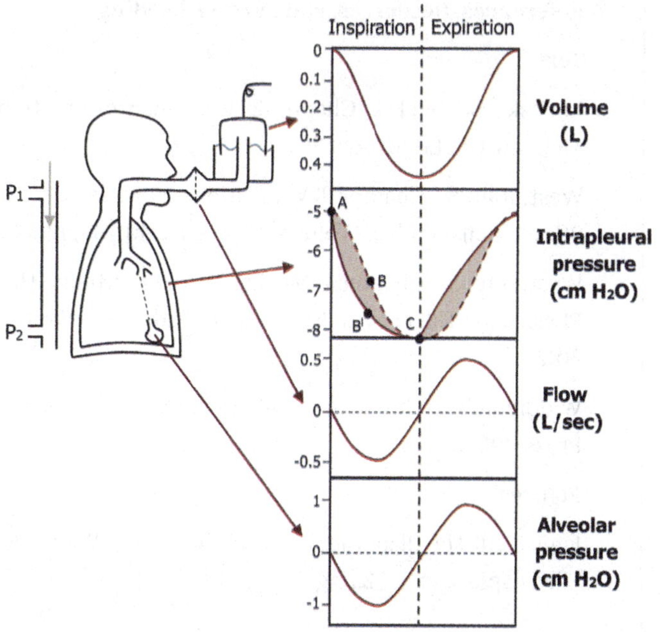

Figure 2.6: The breathing cycle.

Look at what happens (figure 2.6) when the respiratory muscles are activated to increase thoracic volume and achieve a breath in. As the thoracic wall moves outward and the diaphragm descends, thoracic volume and therefore lung volume increases. More tension is generated in the stretching elastic tissue of the lungs as the lung expands—and just like stretching an elastic band, the recoil force increases, and the stretching lung now pulls back harder on the pleural space. This causes the intrapleural pressure to become even more negative (−8 cm H_2O).

This increase in lung volume (and referring back to Boyle's law, the pressure of a gas tends to decrease as the volume of the container increases) causes a decrease in pressure in the lung. This is reflected in a decrease in alveolar pressure.

This drop in alveolar pressure generates a pressure differential between the airways and the atmosphere outside—the atmospheric pressure now being greater than the reduced airway pressure causes the flow of air into the airways and toward the alveoli.

Now let us look at these pressures during expiration. At the end of inspiration the lungs are stretched and the recoil force is high. When the activity of the inspiratory muscles stops, the recoil of the lung is unopposed and the lung recoils (a little like letting go of that stretched elastic band). Therefore, in quiet breathing, the process of breathing out is normally passive and relies on the potential energy stored in the lungs' elastic tissue.

As the lung recoils and returns toward its resting position, the intrapleural pressure becomes less negative and the volume decreases, resulting in a rise in alveolar pressure, as described by Boyle's law. This rise in alveolar pressure means the pressure gradient is reversed, with pressure inside the lung becoming greater than atmospheric pressure. This reversed pressure differential causes the flow of air from the airways toward the outside—and expiration is achieved.

As already mentioned, this is a passive process that relies on lung recoil, and the expiratory muscles remain inactive during quiet breathing. However, when there is a greater ventilatory demand, such as during exercise or lung disease, the respiratory system cannot wait for this passive and relatively slow process to occur, so the expiratory muscles are activated and thoracic volume (and therefore lung volume) is reduced actively much more quickly; this may cause intrapleural pressure to go positive as the thoracic wall actively pushes on the intrapleural space (and the lungs). This positive pleural pressure during active expiration can have significant ramifications in diseased lungs that we will see later on.

References, Resources, and Further Reading

Text

Levitsky, Michael G. "Chapter 2: Mechanics of Breathing." In *Pulmonary Physiology*, 9th ed. New York: McGraw Hill Education, 2018.

West, John B. "Chapter 2: Ventilation—How Gas Gets to the Alveoli." In *Respiratory Physiology: The Essentials*, 9th ed. Philadelphia: Wolters Kluwer Health/Lippincott Williams and Wilkins, 2012.

West, John B. "Chapter 7: Mechanics of Breathing—How the Lung Is Supported and Moved." In *Respiratory Physiology: The Essentials*, 9th ed. Philadelphia: Wolters Kluwer Health/Lippincott Williams and Wilkins, 2012.

Widdicombe, John G., and Andrew S. Davis. "Chapter 1." In *Respiratory Physiology*. Baltimore: University Park Press, 1983.

Figures

Figure 2.1: The diaphragm. Gray, Henry. 1918. Public domain. https://commons.wikimedia.org/wiki/File:Diaphragm_-_2.png

Figure 2.2: Diaphragm positional change. Grey, Kindred. 2022. CC BY 4.0. https://archive.org/details/2.2_20220125

Figure 2.3: Inspiratory muscles of the rib cage. Hafeez, Andeela. 2014. Public domain. https://www.physio-pedia.com/File:949_937_muscles-of-respiration.jpg

Figure 2.4: Expiratory muscles. Hafeez, Andeela. 2014. Public domain. https://www.physio-pedia.com/File:949_937_muscles-of-respiration.jpg

Figure 2.5: The pleural membranes and space. Grey, Kindred. 2022. CC BY 4.0. https://archive.org/details/2.5_20220125

Figure 2.6: The breathing cycle. Grey, Kindred. 2022. CC BY 4.0. https://archive.org/details/2.6_20220125

3. Lung Volumes and Compliance

Learning objectives

- Describe the lung volumes that can be determined by spirometry.
- Describe the factors that determine lung compliance as the lung inflates from residual volume to total lung capacity.
- Describe the ramifications of dead space on the pattern of breathing during hyperpnea.

Lung Volumes

Introduction

In this section we will look at some of the nomenclature for a variety of lung volumes and how these are clinically pertinent and can change in disease. We will also begin to look at the work of breathing and what factors affect how easy or hard the lung is to inflate, that is, lung compliance. We will then see how breathing pattern is generated to improve the efficiency of the lung and reduce the work of breathing.

Lung Volumes

First let us look at lung volumes. This trace from a spirometer (figure 3.1) shows the change in lung volume as a patient breathes normally and then performs some specific maneuvers.

Let us work through the trace from left to right. The initial part of the trace shows resting or "tidal" breathing. The amount of volume inspired during each breath is referred to as **tidal volume**.

Once a normal expiration is complete, however, the lung is far from empty, and when instructed, this patient (figure 3.1) breathes out as far as they can; this excess that comes out the lung is referred to as the **expiratory reserve volume**.

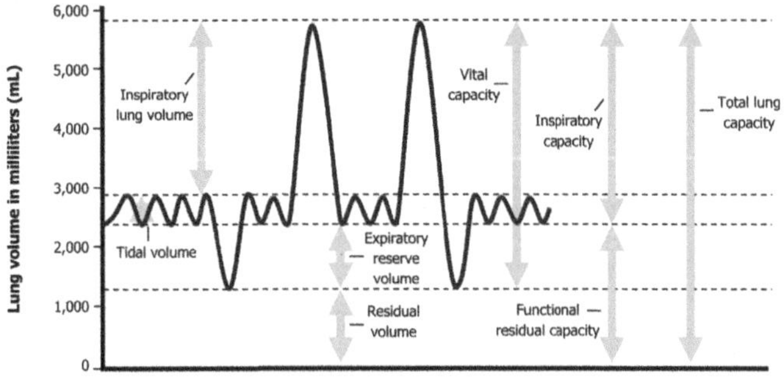

Figure 3.1: Lung volumes detected by spirometry.

Even at this point, however, some air remains in the lung, and this is referred to as **residual volume**. Even with maximal efforts, this volume cannot be exhaled, so at no point can the lung be fully emptied. This also means that residual volume can never be measured with a spirometer.

Our patient (figure 3.1) returns to normal tidal breathing for two breaths before taking a full breath in, filling the lungs as much as they can. This extra volume into the lung after a normal tidal inspiration is referred to as **inspiratory reserve volume**. Related to this volume is the inspiratory capacity, which is the volume that can be taken into the lung after a normal expiration; inspiratory capacity is a useful clinical measurement that we will return to when we deal with some disease states.

Another clinically valuable measurement is **vital capacity**, which is the volume of air that our patient can move out of the lung after a full inspiration, that is, the **total lung capacity**, minus the residual volume (remember: residual volume cannot be expelled). **Forced vital capacity** is a common measure taken in pulmonary function testing, and this is simply the volume that can be expelled from total lung capacity during a forceful expiration. The importance of this maneuver being forced will be dealt with when we look at airway compression (chapter 6).

While the volumes we have just seen measured by spirometry in the pulmonary function lab provide valuable clinical information, we need to now look at some physiological variables that are also critical for our understanding of lung function and disease.

Components of Tidal Breathing

As you have seen, the volume of air inspired during a normal breath is tidal volume, and the size of this is dependent on body size, but in the example here is listed as 500 mL (a good approximation). Not all this 500 mL reaches the gas exchange surfaces in the respiratory zone, however, as some never gets further than the conducting zone (i.e., it stays in the anatomical dead space). From chapter 1 we know that this dead space has a volume of 150 mL, so the amount of air reaching the alveoli in the respiratory zone is our tidal volume (500 mL), minus the dead space volume, so alveolar volume is 350 mL.

This brings us to an important point of clarification. Minute ventilation (denoted as Ve) is the volume of air exchanged in the lung within a minute. This is analogous to cardiac output, the volume of blood pumped by the heart in a minute. As such, minute ventilation is the average tidal volume (V_T) multiplied by the number of breaths taken in a minute (RR).

Equation 3.1

$$Ve = RR \times V_T$$

So if respiratory rate is 10 bpm and tidal volume is 500 mL, minute ventilation is 5,000 mL.

Equation 3.2

$$Ve = 10\,bpm \times 500\,mL = 5,000\,mL\,per\,min$$

Physiologically more important, however, is the alveolar minute ventilation (V_A) that accounts for the "wasted" ventilation that never reached a gas exchange surface but remained in the anatomical dead space. So the calculation for VA is

Equation 3.3

$$V_A = RR \times (V_T - V_D)$$

where V_D is the anatomical dead space (approximately 150 mL). So for our previous example, alveolar minute ventilation is

Equation 3.4

$$V_A = 10 \times (500 - 150\, mL) = 3,500\, mL\, per\, min$$

describing *only* the volume of air that reached the respiratory zone.

So far the involvement of anatomical dead space might seem academic, as it remains constant. But let us consider a different breathing pattern (as often occurs in disease states).

In our example above minute ventilation is 5,000 mL, but accounting for dead space we see that alveolar minute ventilation is 3,500 mL. Now let us consider another breathing pattern—one typical of a patient with restrictive lung disease where tidal volume is reduced and respiratory rate is increased. With a tidal volume of 250 mL and rate of 20, the minute ventilation remains the same, 5,000 mL.

Equation 3.5

$$Ve = 20\, bpm \times 250\, mL = 5,000\, mL\, per\, min$$

But calculating alveolar minute ventilation we see that a greater proportion of the reduced tidal volume is consumed by dead space.

Equation 3.6

$$V_A = 20 \times (250 - 150\, mL) = 2,000\, mL\, per\, min$$

So despite maintaining the same minute ventilation, the second patient's alveolar minute ventilation is reduced by 1,500 mL, which is significant given that this is the volume of air going to the gas exchange surfaces.

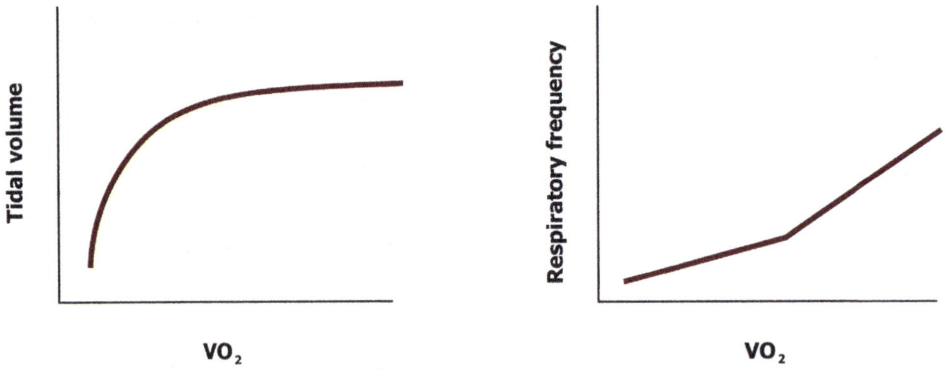

Figure 3.2: Changes in breathing tidal volume and respiratory rate with increasing levels of exercise.

This partially explains why increases in ventilation are initially achieved by increases in tidal volume; as shown in figure 3.2, as tidal volume increases during exercise intensity (represented by oxygen uptake) until it reaches a plateau. Only when this plateau is reached are further increases in minute ventilation achieved by increasing respiratory rate.

So why not keep increasing tidal volume? At higher lung volumes the elastic limit of the lung is approached, and it takes more energy (muscular force) to expand, so it is more efficient and the work of breathing is less if the rate of breathing is increased to achieve higher levels of minute ventilation. This brings us to our next topic, lung compliance.

Lung Compliance

Introduction

Lung compliance is a description of how easy the lung is to inflate, more specifically, how much volume will change for a given pressure differential. Figure 3.3 shows a typical and normal lung compliance curve. The lower line shows how volume changes as intrapleural pressure becomes more negative (as the chest wall and diaphragm expand the thorax). The upper curve is the compliance of the lung during expiration, and it is clearly different; this is an example of hysteresis, meaning that the relationship depends on direction, and we will see why this exists later.

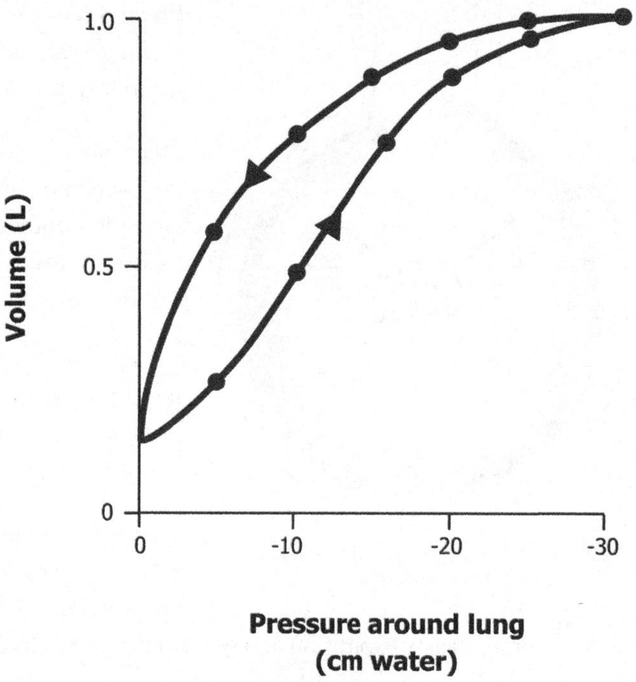

Figure 3.3: Lung compliance curve.

Lung Compliance During Inspiration

You will notice at low lung volumes the slope of the compliance curve (figure 3.3) is shallower, meaning that it takes a relatively large pressure change to cause an increase in volume. This tells us at low lung volumes the lung is less distensible, or has low compliance.

If we start to breathe at a higher lung volume, the slope of the curve is steeper, meaning that for a similar change in pressure there is a greater change in volume (i.e., the lung is more compliant).

If we start breathing at a higher lung volume still, closer to total lung capacity, we see the slope of the compliance curve flatten out again, showing that at the lung volumes the compliance of the lung is low.

As you might imagine, the normal range for breathing is in the middle range where the slope is steep and the lung compliant. This corresponds to an intrapleural pressure range of −5 to −10 cm H_2O, which you should know is the normal range of intrapleural pressures during tidal breathing. This means we normally breathe at a lung volume at which the lung is most compliant and therefore takes less work to inflate.

Too low a lung volume and compliance falls and work of breathing increases, likewise during breathing at high lung volumes, another contributing reason for why tidal volume plateaus during exercise.

So now let us look at why compliance is low at high and low lung volumes, starting with the cause of low lung compliance at low volumes.

Low compliance at low volumes—Surface tension: The reason why the lung takes more pressure to inflate at low volumes is surface tension. As mentioned in chapter 1 the alveoli have a thin layer of fluid lining their inner surface. As we saw in the pleural space, this causes surface tension. Unlike the surface tension in the pleural space, in the alveoli surface tension is a disadvantage.

Surface tension is generated as water molecules cluster together to reduce their exposure to the gas in the alveolar space. As they gather together they drag the alveolar wall with them, producing a force that tends to pull the alveolar walls inward. The alveolar pressure opposes this force and should prevent the alveolus from collapsing (figure 3.4).

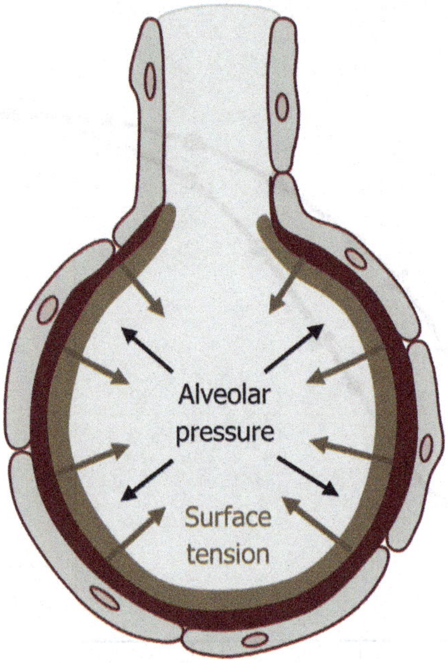

Figure 3.4: Opposing forces of alveolar pressure and surface tension.

The relationship between these two opposing forces is described by Laplace's law that states the outward (alveolar) pressure needed to oppose the inwardly directed tension is proportionate to the tension (obviously), but also inversely related to the radius of the alveolus (i.e., the smaller the radius, the greater the inwardly acting force).

This explains why compliance is low at low lung volumes. At low lung volumes the alveoli are smaller and thus have a smaller radius. Laplace's law states that with a low radius the pressure needed to overcome the inward force will be greater, explaining why a larger alveolar (outward) pressure is needed to inflate the alveolus from a low starting volume.

As lung volume increases, and thus alveolar radius increases, the pressure needed to overcome the inward acting force becomes less and the compliance of the lung increases. This explains why compliance is improved at the normal operating range of lung volumes.

This also explains the hysteresis of the compliance curve. During expiration as alveoli are becoming progressively smaller, the inwardly acting force generated by surface tension becomes progressively greater. This phenomenon consequently assists expiration and contributes to expiration being a passive process.

Low compliance at high lung volumes—Elastic limit: At high lung volumes the alveolar radius has increased further, suggesting that compliance should be further improved as the effect of surface tension will be much less. But surface tension is not the only factor involved, and the compliance curve flattens here, meaning a greater pressure is needed to achieve a volume change at high lung volumes. The low compliance at high lung volumes is caused by another phenomenon altogether. At high lung volumes expansion of the lung becomes limited by the elastic limit of the lung, a little like trying to further stretched an already stretch elastic band—it is harder to do.

So with surface tension causing problems at low lung volumes and tissue elastic limit causing problems at high lung volumes, the compliance curve is steepest (i.e., most favorable) in the middle, as mentioned before, which is the operating volume of the lung. These principles are summarized in figure 3.5.

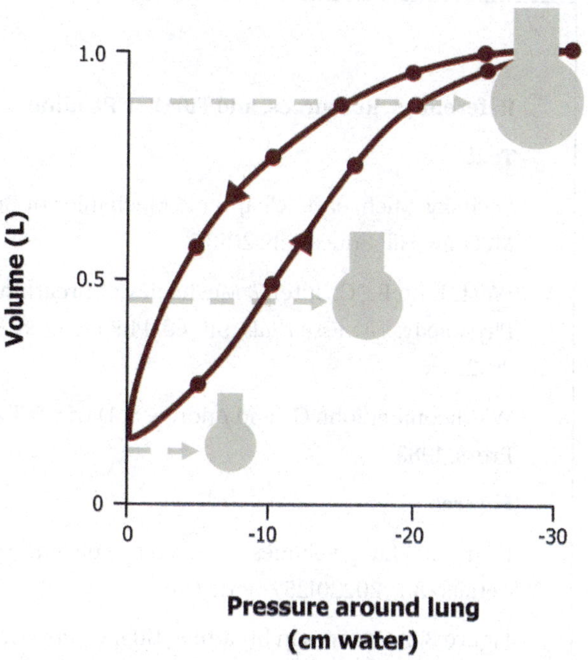

Figure 3.5: Summary of lung volumes and compliance. At low volumes alveoli are small and subject to greater surface tension forces that generate an inwardly acting force that requires greater alveolar pressure to achieve inflation. At higher lung volumes surface tension is less effective at generating an inward force, so less pressure is required to cause inflation (the lung is more compliant). At very high lung volumes surface tension poses even less of a problem, but the elastic limits of the lung are being reached, and increases in volume require alveolar pressures to overcome elastic recoil.

Improving lung compliance with surfactant: So after that information on how surface tension is a problem for the lung, we now have to look at how it could be so much worse if the lung did not protect itself.

Despite it having an effect, particularly at low lung volumes, the lung actually reduces the effect of alveolar surface tension by releasing "surfactant," a molecule that disrupts surface tension. In brief, the surfactant molecule (dipalmitoyl phosphatidylcholine) has a similar structure to the phospholipids that make up cell membranes with a hydrophobic end and a hydrophilic end, allowing it to surround water and repel it at the same time, thus breaking up the interaction between water molecules. So as surfactant significantly reduces surface tension, it thereby increases lung compliance and the risk of alveolar collapse. It also helps keep the air space dry, as excessive surface tension tends to draw water into the space from the capillaries and interstitial spaces.

Surfactant is released onto the alveolar inner surface by Type II alveolar cells (recall Type I cells are those making up the alveolar wall). Type II cells produce surfactant at a high rate and thus demand a constant and generous blood flow; therefore any condition that disrupts this blood supply will cause surfactant concentrations to decline and therefore put the alveolus at risk of collapse as surface tension is allowed to increase.

A good illustration of the effect of surfactant is respiratory distress syndrome of the newborn. The underdeveloped lungs of infants born prematurely (at about twenty-eight weeks), cannot produce sufficient surfactant. Alveoli rapidly collapse (known as atelectasis), and pulmonary edema develops because of the excessive surface tension in the alveolar walls.

References, Resources, and Further Reading

Text

Levitsky, Michael G. "Chapter 2: Mechanics of Breathing." In *Pulmonary Physiology*, 9th ed. New York: McGraw Hill Education, 2018.

West, John B. "Chapter 7: Mechanics of Breathing—How the Lung Is Supported and Moved." In *Respiratory Physiology: The Essentials*, 9th ed. Philadelphia: Wolters Kluwer Health/Lippincott Williams and Wilkins, 2012.

Widdicombe, John G., and Andrew S. Davis. "Chapter 2." In *Respiratory Physiology*. Baltimore: University Park Press, 1983.

Figures

Figure 3.1: Lung volumes detected by spirometry. Grey, Kindred. 2022. CC BY 4.0. https://archive.org/details/3.1_20220125/mode/1up

Figure 3.2: Changes in breathing tidal volume and respiratory rate with increasing levels of exercise. Grey, Kindred. 2022. CC BY 4.0. https://archive.org/details/3.2_20220125/mode/1up

Figure 3.3: Lung compliance curve. Grey, Kindred. 2022. CC BY 4.0. https://archive.org/details/3.3_20220125/mode/1up

Figure 3.4: Opposing forces of alveolar pressure and surface tension. Grey, Kindred. 2022. CC BY 4.0. https://archive.org/details/3.4_20220125/mode/1up

Figure 3.5: Summary of lung volumes and compliance. Grey, Kindred. 2022. CC BY 4.0. https://archive.org/details/3.5_20220125/mode/1up

4. Distribution of Ventilation

Learning objectives

- Describe the distribution of ventilation and how it is affected by gravity and lung volume.

Radial Traction

Introduction

Taking a breath in one might imagine that each part of the lung gets an equal share of the inspired air. But regions of the lung are not equally ventilated. The unequal distribution is caused by (1) gravity and (2) lung volume.

Lung Parenchyma and Radial Traction

Before we look at ventilation distribution we need to understand a little more about lung structure. Although the lung is composed of individual components, such as the alveoli within distinct ascini, the airways, and the blood vessels, the parenchymal tissue between these components helps form the mechanical structure of the lung.

In brief, collagenous and elastic fibers run the length of the large airways and into the lobes forming the axial network. Fibers beneath the pleura and within the septal spaces between the lobes form a peripheral network, and finally thin fibers surrounding the alveoli within the lobes form the septal network. Together these networks form a fibrous "web" of the lung (figure 4.1).

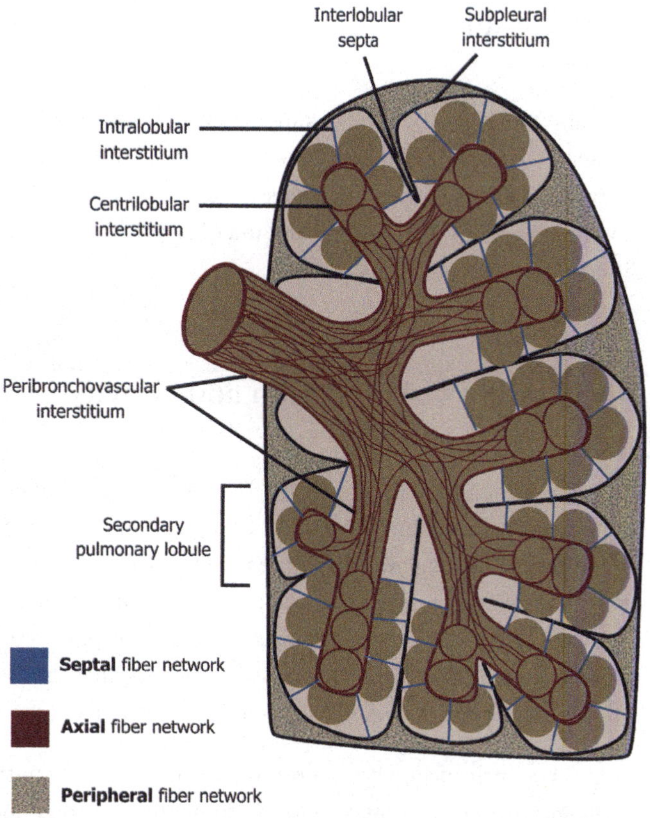

Figure 4.1: The fiber networks of the lung.

Functionally what this means is that movement of one lung structure is transferred to others. As the lung inflates these fibrous connections have a significant impact on lung function and the pulmonary vasculature. Expanding alveoli pull on fibers that are attached to neighboring airways and blood vessels and, indeed, other alveoli.

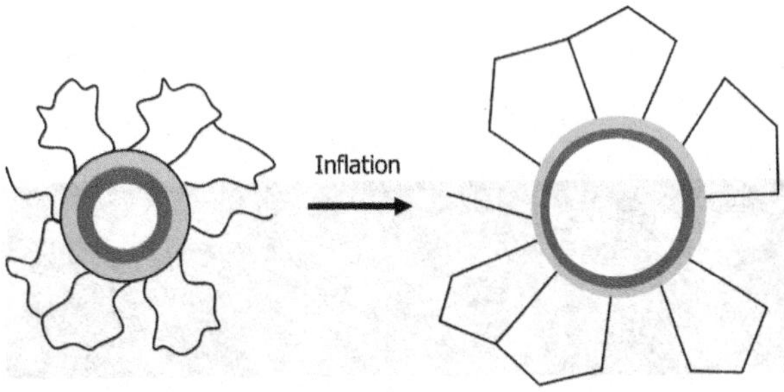

Figure 4.2: The action of radial traction.

The expanding lung volume tends to pull open airways and blood vessels, lowering the resistance of both as inspiration continues, as is illustrated in figure 4.2.

Radial traction (sometimes called parenchymal traction) is an important component of the lung's mechanical behavior, and it means that lung volume has an effect on airway and vascular resistance.

More important for us now though is the understanding that the lung is highly connected within itself. And it is a good thing that it is these fiber networks transfer changes in pleural pressure from the lung periphery to its center; without the networks, only the alveoli at the periphery of the lung would expand when pleural pressure became negative during inspiration.

It also means that the effects of gravity are transferred to the lung as a single unit, and we will look at that now.

Distribution of Ventilation Across the Lung

Introduction

The lung hangs in the thorax supported by the trachea and the surface tension adhering its outer surface to the inside of the thoracic cavity. Gravity obviously tends to pull the lung downward, and this pull has an unequal effect on alveoli at different heights of the lung.

Distribution of Ventilation and Gravity

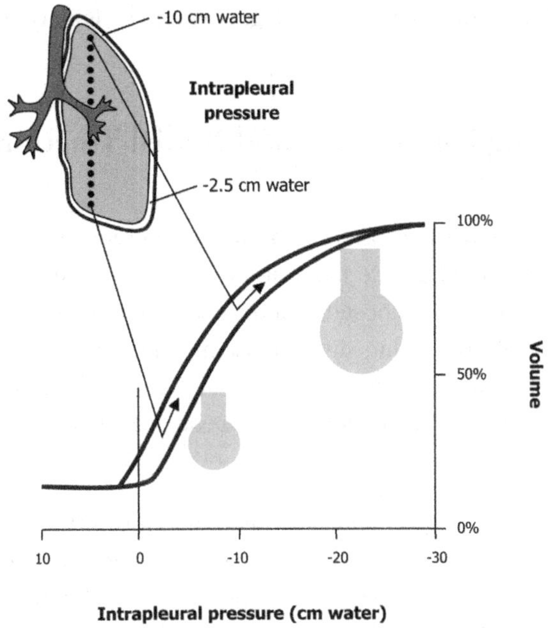

Figure 4.3: Interaction of lung volume, compliance, and distribution of ventilation.

Alveoli at the apex (top) of the lung have a substantial amount of lung tissue below them for gravity to act on, so there is a large force pulling the lung away from the pleural space here and hence at the top of the lung intrapleural pressure is more negative. As we descend down the lung the mass below each point becomes less and less, so the pull on the pleural space declines, and we see intrapleural pressure become less and less negative.

Simply because of gravity, therefore, we have a distribution of intrapleural pressures. As you know from the previous chapter, intrapleural pressure determines alveolus size (figure 4.3). So at the apex of the lung alveoli tend to be large because of the more negative intrapleural pressure, while at the base, alveoli are less extended because of the less negative intrapleural pressure. If an analogy would help, look at this slinky being held up (figure 4.4). The coils near the top of it are pulled far apart because of the weight of the slinky below the top. As you travel down the slinky the coils are less and less extended as less and less weight below pulls on them. The lung acts just the same; alveoli at the top are extended at rest, while those at the base have a smaller volume.

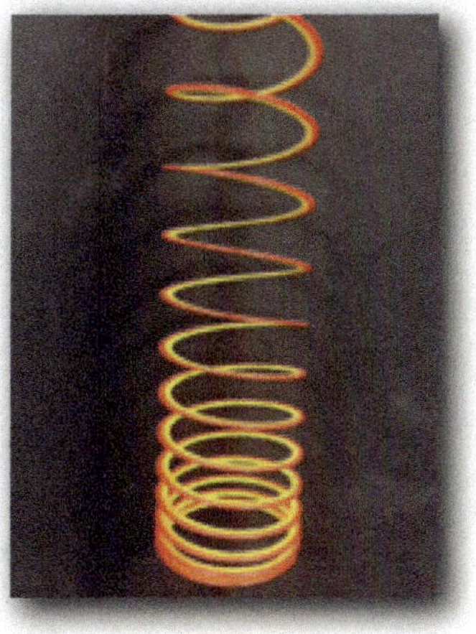

Figure 4.4: Lung = slinky. The weight pulling the coils open becomes less further down the slinky, so the distance between the coils is less nearer the bottom. Gravity acts similarly on the resting lung; with less weight below the alveoli near the base, there is less force pulling the alveoli there open, and the basilar alveoli are smaller than those at the apex.

This has ramifications on where air entering the lung goes and how ventilation is distributed across the lung (more on the implications of this in chapter 13). Alveoli at the apex of the lung are already extended and therefore have limited capacity to take in more air; their resting volume is also close to the flat part of the compliance curve (figure 4.3), so they are more difficult to inflate. The smaller alveoli at the base of the lung, however, still have a greater capacity for expansion, and the smaller resting volume places them on the steeper section of the compliance curve; consequently they are easier to inflate, and air takes the path of least resistance.

Because of this, the alveoli at the apex of the lung rapidly fill to capacity on inspiration, and the vast majority of inspired air descends toward the base toward the more compliant and less extended alveoli. This uneven distribution of ventilation is something we will return to when we address other learning objectives, so it is worth understanding.

Distribution of Ventilation and Lung Volume

The distribution of ventilation is also effected by lung volume, and at low lung volumes the apex of the lung is actually better ventilated than the base—again, this is due to changes in alveolar compliance.

As the lung is emptied below functional residual capacity, that is below the normal point that expiration ends, the recoil of the lung is reduced and therefore intrapleural pressure becomes progressively less negative (or more positive if that is the way you would like to think of it). Compared to the normal resting volume we just dealt with, at low lung volumes the intrapleural pressure may be up to −4 cm H_2O (compared to −10). This pushes the apical alveoli down on to the steep part of the compliance curve, and therefore they are easier to inflate.

The intrapleural pressure at the base of the lung may actually become positive at low lung volumes. Now that force that tended to open up alveoli is actually a force that tends to compress alveoli. In our example here the intrapleural reaches 3.5 cm H_2O, a force that may lead to airway compression and thereby reduce ventilation to the basal alveoli. This intrapleural pressure will certainly place these alveoli on the very flat and therefore noncompliant section of the compliance curve and make them difficult to inflate because of the surface tension and small radius effect we have discussed previously.

Summary

Ventilation is unevenly distributed across the lung because of the range of intrapleural pressures that are established down the lung by gravity. At normal lung volumes the base of the lung is better ventilated than the apex.

At low lung volumes this relationship is reversed as intrapleural pressures at the base of the lung become compressive, reducing the compliance of basal alveoli, while the compliance of apical alveoli is increased.

References, Resources, and Further Reading

Text

Levitsky, Michael G. "Chapter 2: Mechanics of Breathing." In *Pulmonary Physiology*, 9th ed. New York: McGraw Hill Education, 2018.

West, John B. "Chapter 7: Mechanics of Breathing—How the Lung Is Supported and Moved." In *Respiratory Physiology: The Essentials*, 9th ed. Philadelphia: Wolters Kluwer Health/Lippincott Williams and Wilkins, 2012.

Widdicombe, John G., and Andrew S. Davis. "Chapter 1." In *Respiratory Physiology*. Baltimore: University Park Press, 1983.

Figures

Figure 4.1: The fiber networks of the lung. Grey, Kindred. 2022. CC BY 4.0. https://archive.org/details/4.1_20220125/mode/1up

Figure 4.2: The action of radial traction. Grey, Kindred. 2022. CC BY 4.0. https://archive.org/details/4.2_20220125/mode/1up

Figure 4.3: Interaction of lung volume, compliance, and distribution of ventilation. Grey, Kindred. 2022. CC BY 4.0. https://archive.org/details/4.3_20220125/mode/1up

Figure 4.4: Lung = slinky. Binks, Andrew. 2022. CC BY-NC-SA 4.0.

5. Airflow and Airway Resistance

Learning objectives

- Describe the factors that contribute to airway resistance.
- Describe the changes in airway resistance down the bronchial tree, with expanding lung volumes and induced by autonomic reflexes.

Fundamentals of Airflow

To generate flow in the airways, so far we have looked at how the pressure differential is generated and the factors affecting the compliance of the lung. Now we will look at the factors that cause resistance to airflow and how mechanical and neural influences affect it.

The first factor we must consider when thinking about airflow is the type of flow that is occurring.

The most efficient form of flow is laminar (i.e., laminar flow takes the lowest pressure differential for flow to occur). In laminar flow the molecules are moving in an orderly manner, those at the side of the tube moving a little slower due to contact with tube walls and those in the middle moving fastest (figure 5.1).

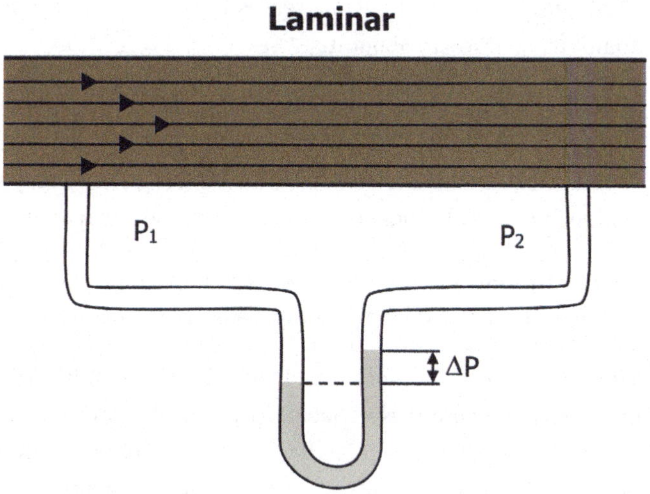

Figure 5.1: Laminar flow.

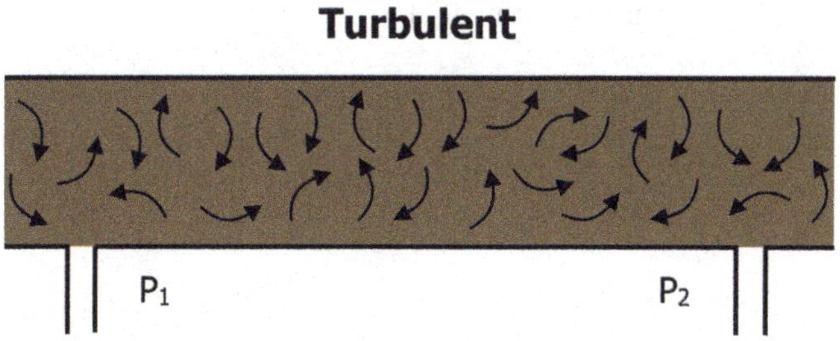

Figure 5.2: Turbulent flow.

When velocity increases or tube radius decreases then this organization is lost. Collisions between molecules and with the tube wall are now more frequent and movement is more chaotic, and the flow becomes turbulent (figure 5.2). At this point some molecules are at times moving against the pressure gradient due to these collisions. Consequently, to generate the same amount of molecule movement (i.e., flow) from one end of the tube to another, a greater pressure differential is needed when flow becomes turbulent. Turbulent flow is more common in the large airways where velocity and airway radius are high.

In reality, the vast majority of the airways are branching small tubes, so we see a mixture of the two above—mostly laminar flow but some turbulence generated at the branch (or transitional) points (figure 5.3).

For our purposes though we are going to look at the factors that affect flow when it is laminar—the dominant form of flow in the majority of airways. These factors are described by Poiselle's equation. We will now break down Poiselle's equation in relation to flow of air down airways. Although initially an intimidating equation, there are some things we can generally ignore.

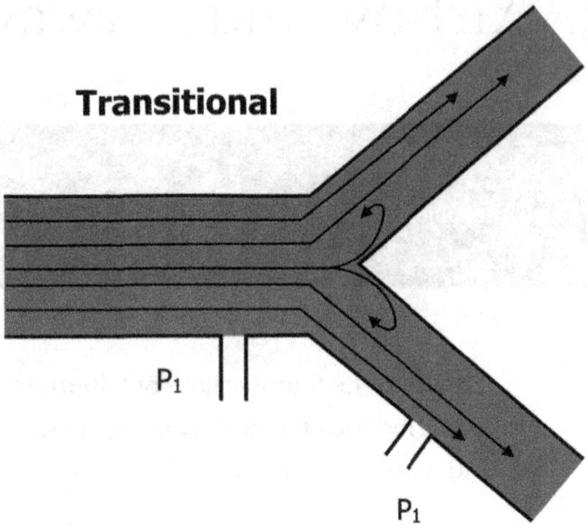

Figure 5.3: Transitional flow.

Equation 5.1

$$\dot{V} = \frac{\Delta P \times \pi \times r^4}{8n \times L}$$

First, Poiselle says that flow increases when length of the tube increases; because the airways have constant length, we do not have to worry about it.

Then there is the viscosity of the gas. This is not usually a concern either when breathing humidified air at a constant biological temperature. It does become important when breathing other gas mixtures, however, such as a helium/oxygen blend that has a lower viscosity and is given to respiratory patients or deep water divers to increase flow. But we will assume it is another constant. Pi (π) is also a constant.

So the two remaining variables are the important ones to understand. The pressure differential created by expansion and relaxation of the lung generates a proportional flow, and we have dealt with this in previous chapters.

What we will look at more closely now is airway radius as this has a profound effect on flow. Radius is critical for two main reasons. First it is variable, as the caliber of an airway changes with lung volume and by the action of airway smooth muscle. Second, it has a very powerful effect on flow; as you can see in Poiselle's equation, radius is to the fourth power. This means a small increase in radius has a large effect on flow. For example, if the radius of an airway is doubled from 1 mm to 2 mm, the flow rate through the tube increases sixteenfold, which of course is two to the fourth power (i.e., 2x2x2x2). The inverse is of course true—halve the radius and flow reduces sixteenfold.

So far we have couched everything in terms of flow, but really we need to look at airway resistance. Because resistance is simply the reciprocal (or opposite) of flow, we can flip Poiselle's equation upside down to describe resistance, and we now see that a reduction in radius (r) causes a large increase in resistance (R).

Equation 5.2

$$R = \frac{8n \times L}{\Delta P \times \pi \times r^4}$$

Airway Resistance

So with radius having such a powerful effect on airway resistance we would expect that the early and larger generations of airways would offer the least resistance to flow, and resistance would increase as we descended deeper into the lung to the smaller and later airway generations. Figure 5.4 shows the opposite is true—that airway resistance decreases as the airway generations are descended. This is because the total cross-sectional area increases with each generation—while the early and large airways are wide, they are few. The lower and smaller airways are much more numerous, and so collectively they have a greater cross-sectional area and therefore offer less resistance.

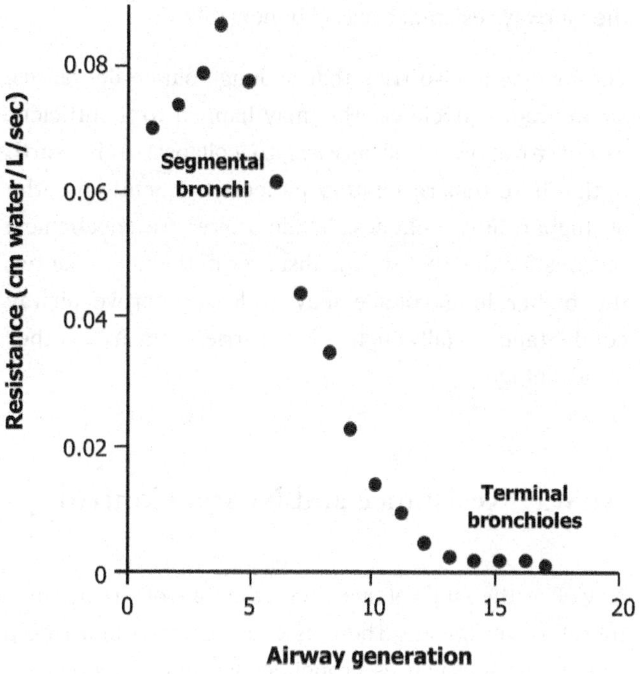

Figure 5.4: Airway resistance down the bronchial tree.

The highest point of resistance is actually the midsize bronchioles. There are a couple of clinically important points to make here:

1. If radius is reduced by disease, such as during inflammation of the airway wall or contraction of airway smooth muscle causing bronchoconstriction, then resistance is markedly increased, and to maintain flow, the pressure differential must be increased. Increasing this pressure differential means increasing the work of breathing.
2. The vast total cross-sectional area of the lower airways means that a significant amount of damage can be done before symptoms arise. This "silent zone" means that a disease may be significantly established and be in a relatively late stage before the patient becomes symptomatic and goes to the physician.

Airway Resistance and Lung Volume

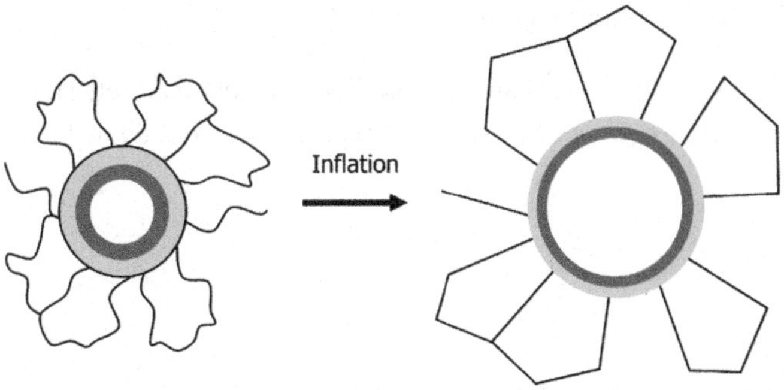

Figure 5.5: Radial traction decreases airway resistance as lung volume increases.

The airways without cartilaginous support significantly change their radius when the lung expands due to the radial traction. In brief, parenchymal fibers tethered to the alveoli and exterior of the airways allow the airways to be pulled open by the expanding alveoli when lung volume increases (illustrated in figure 5.5).

This increase in airway diameter means that airway resistance falls as lung volume increases. This is demonstrated by figure 5.6; as lung volume increases, then airway resistance falls exponentially.

The inverse is also true, that as lung volume decreases, airway radius declines. This may happen to a sufficient extent to allow small airways to collapse. It is worth noting here that respiratory patients frequently breathe at higher lung volumes. While there are mechanical reasons for this that we will discover in the next chapter, the higher lung volume may at least improve airway conductance (although it carries many other disadvantages).

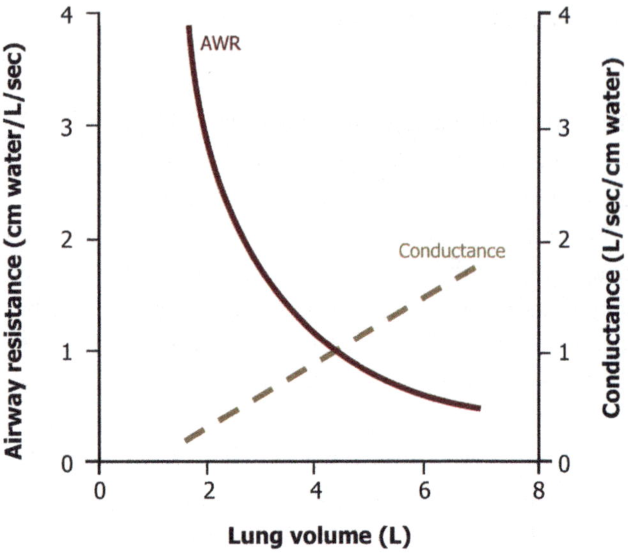

Figure 5.6: Airway resistance and lung volume.

Airway Resistance and Neural Control

As well as the lung volume effect, the tone of airway smooth muscle is also a powerful determinant of airway radius and therefore resistance. The muscle is arranged in a ring pattern around the airway circumference. Contraction of the smooth muscle causes bronchoconstriction, decreasing the airway radius. Relaxation of the smooth muscle allows bronchodilation.

Airway smooth muscle is under the control of the autonomic nervous system. Parasympathetic release of acetylcholine causes activation of muscarinic receptors. This causes a rise in intracellular calcium that activates the smooth muscle. Muscle is relaxed by sympathetic stimulation of β_2 adrenergic receptors. These β_2 receptors are the target of bronchodilator drugs, such as albuterol, that resolve the inappropriate contraction of smooth muscle seen in the hypersensitive airways of asthmatics.

The bronchoconstrictive pathway is utilized by the irritant reflex that is initiated by airway wall receptors detecting the arrival of inspired particulates. This defensive reflex results in bronchoconstriction, presumably to limit the entry of more particulates.

A number of inflammatory mediators also cause bronchoconstriction and probably play a significant role in the bronchoconstriction of asthma (which frequently also involves airway inflammation).

Low airway PCO_2 also has a direct stimulatory effect on airway smooth muscle and a bronchoconstrictive effect. This is presumably to shunt air to other regions of the lung and away from regions where overventilation caused the low PCO_2.

Summary

So now you should be able to understand how the type of flow, airway radius, lung volume, and autonomic nervous system all influence airway resistance and so can either oppose or promote the flow of air in the lung.

References, Resources, and Further Reading

Text

Levitsky, Michael G. "Chapter 2: Mechanics of Breathing." In *Pulmonary Physiology*, 9th ed. New York: McGraw Hill Education, 2018.

West, John B. "Chapter 7: Mechanics of Breathing—How the Lung Is Supported and Moved." In *Respiratory Physiology: The Essentials*, 9th ed. Philadelphia: Wolters Kluwer Health/Lippincott Williams and Wilkins, 2012.

Widdicombe, John G., and Andrew S. Davis. "Chapter 3." In *Respiratory Physiology*. Baltimore: University Park Press, 1983.

Figures

Figure 5.1: Laminar flow. Grey, Kindred. 2022. CC BY 4.0. https://archive.org/details/5.1_20220125/mode/1up

Figure 5.2: Turbulent flow. Grey, Kindred. 2022. CC BY 4.0. https://archive.org/details/5.2_20220125/mode/1up

Figure 5.3: Transitional flow. Grey, Kindred. 2022. CC BY 4.0. https://archive.org/details/5.3_20220125/mode/1up

Figure 5.4: Airway resistance down the bronchial tree. Grey, Kindred. 2022. CC BY 4.0. https://archive.org/details/5.6_20220125/mode/1up

Figure 5.5: Radial traction decreases airway resistance as lung volume increases. Grey, Kindred. 2022. CC BY 4.0. https://archive.org/details/5.7_20220125/mode/1up

Figure 5.6: Airway resistance and lung volume. Grey, Kindred. 2022. CC BY 4.0. https://archive.org/details/5.8_20220125/mode/1up

6. Dynamic Airway Compression

Learning objectives

- Describe how pleural and airway pressures interact to cause dynamic airway compression in the healthy lung and how this is exacerbated in disease.
- Briefly describe how flow-volume loops can help distinguish between obstructive and restrictive lung diseases.

Compression of Airways During Expiration

The interaction of intrapleural and airway pressures is relatively simple during inspiration; intrapleural pressure becomes more negative, and the airways are pulled open as lung volume increases. This chapter will focus on the interaction of these forces during expiration and the potential for intrapleural pressure to cause airway compression.

Although this phenomenon is present in the healthy lung, we will see how it is exacerbated in certain disease states and how this exacerbation can be detected by common pulmonary function tests.

First, let us look at the forces involved during a normal, passive expiration.

For simplicity, the schematic in figure 6.1 shows one airway and an alveolus within the thoracic cavity. At the onset of passive expiration (driven by the recoil of the expanded lung), the intrapleural pressure is negative (about −8 cm H_2O). As it remains negative, intrapleural pressure helps keep the airways open.

The elastic forces of the alveolus wall exert an inward force of about +10 cm H_2O. This results in a net force of +2 cm H_2O in the alveolus, and a gradient between this positive pressure is established between the alveolus and the atmosphere outside the lung. That means that along the airway toward the mouth there is a gradient of progressively decreasing pressure to zero (shown in maroon).

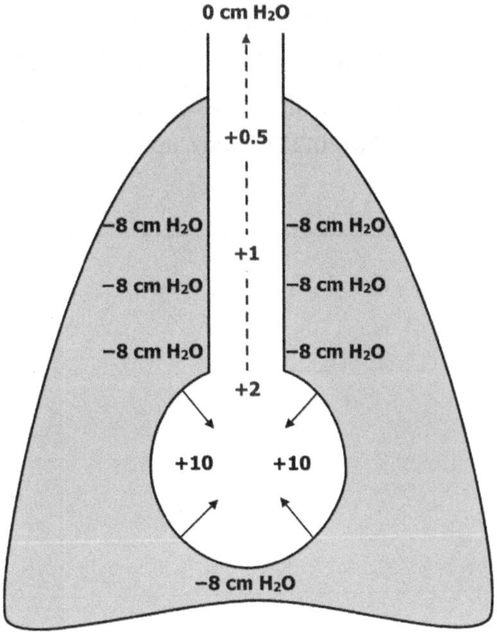

Figure 6.1: Intrapleural and airway pressures during normal/passive expiration.

Importantly in this example of passive expiration the airway pressure is greater than the pleural pressure along the whole length of the airway toward the mouth. Along with the radial traction provided by the surrounding parenchymal tissue, this favorable transmural pressure gradient helps keep the airway open during expiration.

Now let us look at what happens if expiration is forceful, or active, rather than passively relying on lung recoil.

In a forced expiration (see figure 6.2) the intrapleural pressure can become positive (as much as 120 cm H_2O), but in this example we will say it is 25 cm H_2O. This positive pressure in the pleural cavity comes from the chest wall and diaphragm now "pushing" the pleural membranes together and compressing the lung.

Again, we have the elastic forces of the alveolus generating an inward force (still +10 cm H_2O), and when summed with the now positive intrapleural forces, we end up with an alveolar pressure of +35 cm H_2O.

Again, a pressure gradient between the alveolus and the atmosphere is established (again shown in maroon), but this time there is a fundamental difference caused by the larger intrapleural pressure.

At some point along the airway, as airway pressure is decreasing, the intrapleural pressure exceeds airway pressure (in this example it is 25 cm H_2O). At this "choke" point (arrows pointing toward airway in figure 6.2), the airway can become compressed or even collapse.

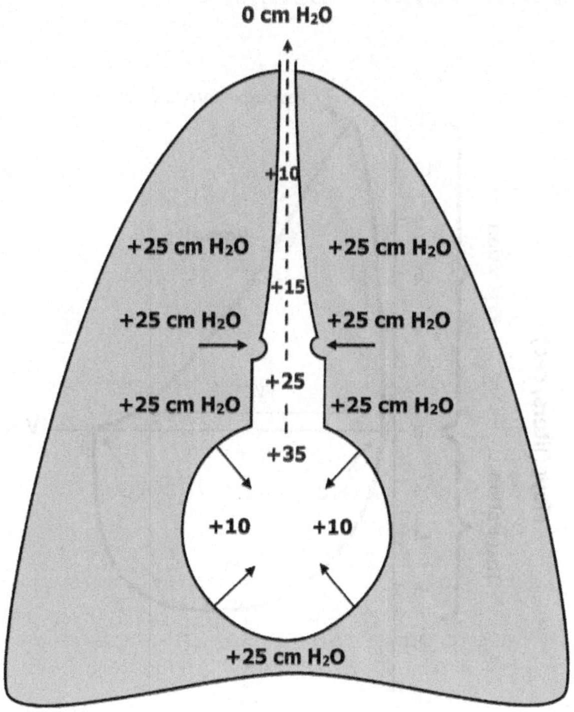

Figure 6.2: Intrapleural and airway pressures during forced expiration.

This effect is somewhat reduced by the radial traction of the parenchyma, but airway compression occurs even in the healthy normal lung, and the greater the effort of expiration (i.e., the more positive the intrapleural pressure), the greater degree airways compress and compression occurs closer to the alveoli (i.e., further up the pressure gradient in the airway).

If airways are already narrowed, as in obstructive lung diseases such as asthma, or parenchymal traction is lost, such as in emphysema, dynamic airway compression occurs to a greater extent. In these obstructive diseases the increased airway resistance results in the patient having to forcefully expire to overcome the increased resistance of the narrowed airways. This promotes airway compression and leads to air being trapped behind the choke point, causing hyperinflation (breathing at an elevated lung volume).

This airway compression or any other increase in airway resistance can be demonstrated by a common pulmonary function test, the flow-volume loop.

Flow-Volume Loops

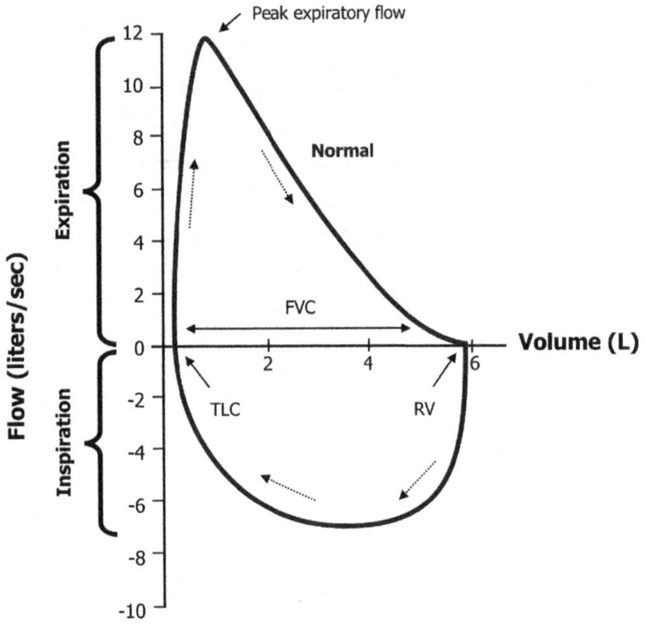

Figure 6.3: Typical and normal flow-volume loop. FVC: forved vital capacity

Flow-volume loops are briefly discussed in context of the relevant physiology. Figure 6.3 shows a normal flow-volume loop. Note that the volume axis seems to be the wrong way around; this is because expired volume and flow are generally more useful, so the plot has expiratory flow as positive and lung volume orientated for expiration. While breathing on a spirometer, the patient begins to breathe in from residual volume (bottom half of maroon line). As inspiration continues, lung volume increases (moves toward the y-axis) and airflow increases (moves downward). The patient continues inhaling until they are at total lung capacity (or TLC).

They then exhale as hard and as fast as they can, forcefully emptying the lung as quickly as possible. During forced exhalation of the first liter or so, expiratory flow rapidly increases until it reaches peak expiratory flow; this is the first clinically pertinent measure. After this point expiratory flow begins an exponential decline; as lung volume continues to decrease, so does the flow rate until flow reaches zero when the lung is emptied (at residual volume).

The rate of this decline in flow rate is also an important clinical measure and brings together a couple of important physiological points:

1. Flow is declining during this phase of expiration due to the forceful expiration causing airway compression and thereby increasing airway resistance.
2. Airways will also become smaller as radial traction of the parenchyma also declines with lung volume.

Although there are a number of measurements that are calculated from this forced exhalation, two are most commonly reported. First, the total volume that is expelled from the lung is referred to as the forced vital capacity (FVC). The forced expiratory volume that is expelled from the lung in the first second of expiration is referred to as FEV_1. The ratio of these two values, known as FEV_1/FVC, describes the percentage of lung volume that can be emptied in one second and is a useful indicator of airway resistance. A normal FEV_1/FVC is 90 percent or higher, meaning over 90 percent of vital capacity can be emptied from the lung within a second. This value is dependent on age, gender, and body size, but commonly used predicted values take these variables into account when assessing for disease.

The loop produced by a patient with chronic obstructive lung disease, or COPD, looks very different (gray line in figure 6.4). With disease causing airway narrowing, the peak expiratory flow is significantly reduced, and the decay in expiratory flow as lung volume declines is much more pronounced as the narrowed airways can be easier to collapse due to a lower starting radius and/or loss of radial traction.

This means that FEV_1 is significantly reduced, but FVC may remain unchanged (i.e., the lung volume is the same, but it takes longer to empty). An FEV_1/FVC significantly less than 90 percent is indicative of obstructive disease. Notice that the inspiratory loop of the COPD patient appears normal, illustrating the effect of increasingly negative intrapleural pressure, increasing lung volume and radial traction on airway resistance.

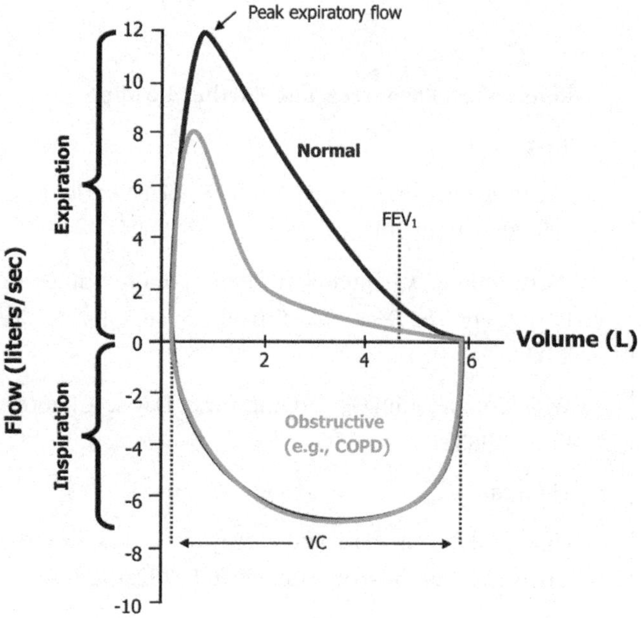

Figure 6.4: Normal (maroon) and obstructive disease (gray) flow-volume loops.

Alternatively, diseases that restrict lung expansion (figure 6.5), such as pulmonary fibrosis, demonstrate a reduced lung volume, where FVC is substantially reduced, but FEV_1 may not be significantly affected; in fact it is not uncommon for FEV_1/FVC to increase to about normal in restricted diseases, but this is of course due to a decline in FVC rather than a rise in FEV_1. Notice also that the inspiratory loop is affected, with volumes being reduced here as well.

A flow-volume loop is a quick, cheap, and powerful diagnostic measure, but it is highly dependent on the patient performing a forced expiration to encourage dynamic compression and peak flows be obtained so that any airway abnormalities can be seen. This is why you may hear a pulmonary function technologist (PFT) shouting encouragement to a patient as you walk past the lab.

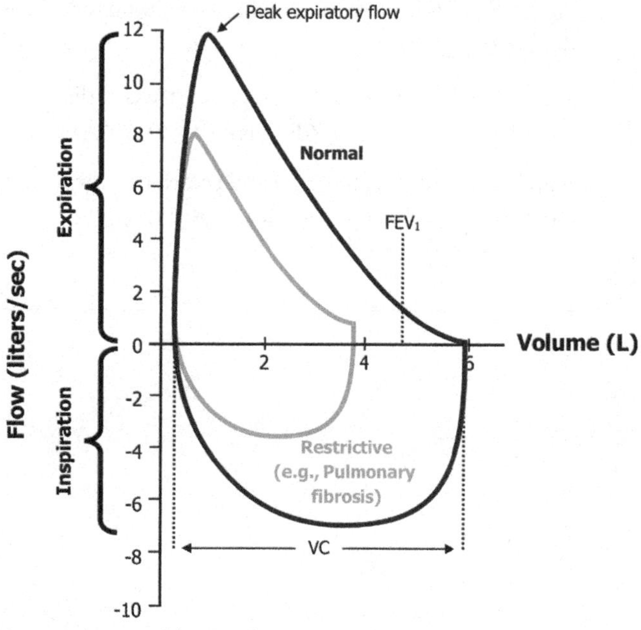

Figure 6.5: Normal (maroon) and restrictive (gray) flow-volume loops.

Summary

So we have dealt with a couple of relatively complex issues in this chapter, particularly the interaction between intrapleural pressure and airway pressure during forced or active expirations and how airways can become compressed.

We have also looked at the use of flow-volume loops to determine the degree of airway obstruction and to distinguish between obstructive and restrictive disorders.

References, Resources, and Further Reading

Text

Levitsky, Michael G. "Chapter 3: Alveolar Ventilation." In *Pulmonary Physiology*, 9th ed. New York: McGraw Hill Education, 2018.

West, John B. "Chapter 7: Mechanics of Breathing—How the Lung Is Supported and Moved." In *Respiratory Physiology: The Essentials*, 9th ed. Philadelphia: Wolters Kluwer Health/Lippincott Williams and Wilkins, 2012.

Widdicombe, John G., and Andrew S. Davis. "Chapter 3." In *Respiratory Physiology*. Baltimore: University Park Press, 1983.

Figures

Figure 6.1: Intrapleural and airway pressures during normal/passive expiration. Grey, Kindred. 2022. CC BY 4.0. https://archive.org/details/6.1_20220125

Figure 6.2: Intrapleural and airway pressures during forced expiration. Grey, Kindred. 2022. CC BY 4.0. https://archive.org/details/6.2_20220125

Figure 6.3: Typical and normal flow-volume loop. Grey, Kindred. 2022. CC BY 4.0. https://archive.org/details/6.3_20220125

Figure 6.4: Normal (maroon) and obstructive disease (gray) flow-volume loops. Grey, Kindred. 2022. CC BY 4.0. https://archive.org/details/6.4_20220125

Figure 6.5: Normal (maroon) and restrictive (gray) flow-volume loops. Grey, Kindred. 2022. CC BY 4.0. https://archive.org/details/6.5_20220125

7. Fundamentals of Gas Exchange

Learning objectives

- Calculate a partial pressure of a gas of known concentration at a known barometric pressure.
- Describe how changes in factors included in Fick's law of diffusion may contribute to incomplete gas exchange.

Partial Pressures

The lung is well designed to perform its function of gas exchange with the atmosphere, and in this chapter we will look at some of the factors that allow the lung to perform this function and how these factors might change in disease.

Before we do that though, we need to be able to calculate the units of measurement we use when describing gas exchange. When referring to gas exchange we are really referring to diffusion of gases down their concentration gradient, but rather than use concentrations, we use partial pressures.

Partial pressures describe what proportion of the total pressure is exerted by a particular component of a mixed gas. Let us look at the specific situation we are interested in to illustrate this description.

Atmospheric pressure at sea level is 760 mmHg. This pressure is generated by the collisions of all the molecules with each other and other objects. At high altitude there are fewer molecules, so fewer collisions, and hence atmospheric pressure is lower.

Now looking at the composition of our atmosphere we know that 79 percent is nitrogen, 20.9 percent is oxygen, and some trace gases collectively get us to 100 percent. Now let us calculate a partial pressure. If 79 percent of the atmosphere is nitrogen, then 79 percent of our atmospheric pressure is generated by the collisions by nitrogen molecules. Likewise 20.9 percent of the atmospheric pressure is due to oxygen, so to calculate the partial pressure of oxygen (PO_2) we simply multiply atmospheric pressure (P_B) by the percentage of oxygen, which means our atmosphere has a partial pressure of oxygen of 159 mmHg.

$$PO_2 = \%O_2 \times P_B$$

$$PO_2 = 20.9\% \times 760\, mmHg = 159\, mmHg$$

Alveolar PO_2

Although related, we are more interested in the PO_2 at the gas exchange surface—that is the alveolar PO_2 denoted as P_AO_2 (note the uppercase A; lowercase refers to arterial PO_2 (i.e., P_aO_2)). This value differs significantly from atmospheric PO_2 at about 100 mmHg. So why the drop of nearly 60 mmHg from atmospheric PO_2?

To calculate alveolar PO_2 we need to account for the water vapor that is added to the inspired air as it enters the airways. This is equivalent to adding another gas and must be accounted for. Water vapor exerts a pressure of 47 mmHg. Subtracting this from our atmospheric pressure, our total gaseous pressure is 713 mmHg; multiplying this by our fraction of inspired O_2 (FiO_2 is merely the percentage (fraction) of oxygen inspired), we see our alveolar PO_2 is theoretically 149.7 mmHg (i.e., ~150 mmHg).

$$P_AO_2 = FiO_2 \times (P_B - P_{H_2O})$$

$$P_AO_2 = 20.9\% \times (760 - 47) = 149.7\, mmHg\, or \sim 150\, mmHg$$

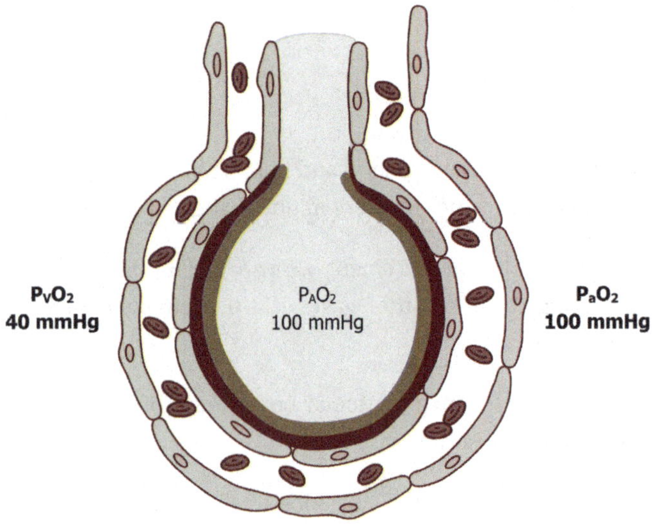

Figure 7.1: Oxygen tensions around the alveolus.

If we understand that there will be mixing with air remaining from the previous breath, the real P_AO_2 is 100 mmHg (however, we will see this varies across the regions of the lung).

So how does this value relate to gas exchange in the lung? The venous blood PO_2 (P_VO_2), returning from the systemic tissue where oxygen has been consumed, is 40 mmHg (see figure 7.1). This blood passes the gas exchange surface, and a pressure gradient of 60 mmHg allows oxygen to move into the pulmonary blood. By the time the blood has passed the alveolus, arterial PO_2 will have equilibrated with the alveolar PO_2 and will also be 100 mmHg. These numbers are well worth committing to memory.

The other critical values we need to address here are the partial pressures of CO_2 (see figure 7.2). Venous blood returning from the tissue has a PCO_2 of 45 mmHg, compared to alveolar PCO_2 that is 40 mmHg. This pressure gradient of 5 mmHg is enough to allow blood to equilibrate with the alveolus, and so arterial PCO_2 is 40 mmHg. Again, these numbers are worth remembering.

A much smaller diffusion gradient is needed for CO_2 because CO_2 is much more soluble than oxygen, a factor among others that is included in Fick's law of diffusion.

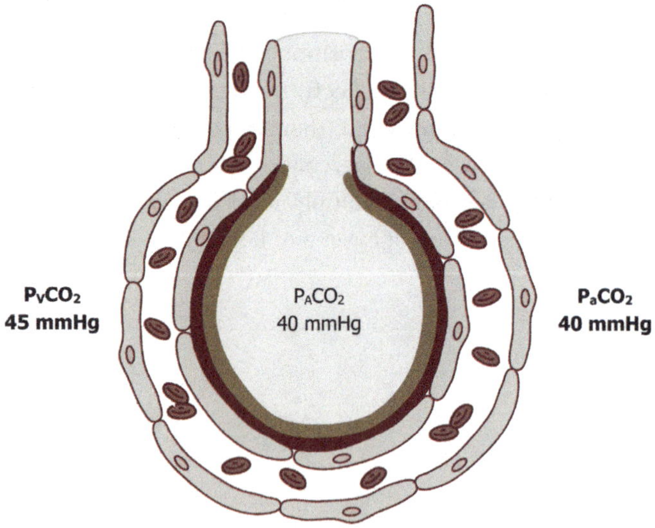

Figure 7.2: Carbon dioxide tensions around the alveolus.

Fick's Law of Diffusion

Fick's law of diffusion (equation 7.1) describes all the factors that influence the transfer of gas (or flow, V) across a membrane.

Equation 7.1

$$\dot{V} \propto \frac{A}{T} \times D \times (P_1 - P_2)$$

We will look at each factor in the equation and see how it relates to the physiology of the lung.

Pressure gradient (P_1–P_2): The higher the pressure gradient, the greater the transfer of gas, and the pressure gradient must be maintained for gas exchange to continue. The maintenance of the gradient is achieved by adequate ventilation to the alveolus to refresh the alveolar gases, and adequate perfusion to flush oxygen away from the gas exchange surface and supply more CO_2. We will look at the importance of matching ventilation and perfusion in chapter 13.

Other factors in Fick's law are fairly obvious and are reflected in the lung's structure.

Surface area (A): The greater the surface area available for exchange, the greater the exchange. The lung has a surface area of 100 m^2, which is more than adequate to maintain sufficient gas transfer, even during maximal exercise.

Membrane thickness (T): The thickness of the membrane that gas has to cross also determines the rate of transfer; the thinner the membrane, the more rapid the transfer. The gas exchange membrane in the lung is approximately a 0.3 um thick—and poses little opposition to gas movement.

Diffusion constant (D): The last variable is the diffusion constant of the gases in question, which for us are O_2 and CO_2. The important issue here is that CO_2 is much more soluble (x 20) than O_2 and so has a much greater diffusion constant; hence it transfers across the membrane much more readily and does not need the large pressure gradient like the relatively insoluble oxygen (5 mmHg compared with 60 mmHg).

Some of these factors can change in lung disease and can result in decreased gas exchange and so result in deranged blood gases. Loss of surface area occurs in diseases, such as emphysema, that destroy the lung architecture, and cause a loss of gas transfer. Likewise, any disease that causes thickening of the alveolar membrane, such as pulmonary fibrosis, increases the distance for, and resistance to, gas transfer. If ventilation or perfusion of the gas exchange surface fails—for example, a mucus plug blocking an airway or a pulmonary embolus blocking a vessel—then the pressure gradient across the membrane is lost and gas exchange is reduced compared to the ideal situation of ventilation and perfusion being matched.

Summary

After this chapter you should be able to calculate the alveolar partial pressure of a gas at any atmospheric pressure and relate it to the rate of gas exchange.

You should also now understand the different factors that contribute to the rate of gas exchange described in Fick's law of diffusion and be able to appreciate how they might change in disease.

References, Resources, and Further Reading

Text

Levitsky, Michael G. "Chapter 6: Diffusion of Gases and Interpretation of Pulmonary Function Tests." In *Pulmonary Physiology*, 9th ed. New York: McGraw Hill Education, 2018.

West, John B. "Chapter 3: Diffusion—How Gas Gets Across the Blood-Gas Barrier." In *Respiratory Physiology: The Essentials*, 9th ed. Philadelphia: Wolters Kluwer Health/Lippincott Williams and Wilkins, 2012.

Widdicombe, John G., and Andrew S. Davis. "Chapter 4." In *Respiratory Physiology*. Baltimore: University Park Press, 1983.

Figures

Figure 7.1: Oxygen tensions around the alveolus. Grey, Kindred. 2022. CC BY 4.0. Added red blood cells by Lucas Helle from Noun Project. CC BY 3.0. https://archive.org/details/7.1_20220125

Figure 7.2: Carbon dioxide tensions around the alveolus. Grey, Kindred. 2022. CC BY 4.0. Added red blood cells by Lucas Helle from Noun Project. CC BY 3.0. https://archive.org/details/7.2_20220125

8. Perfusion and Diffusion Limitations in Gas Exchange

Learning objectives

- Differentiate between diffusion and perfusion limitations to gas exchange and describe the effects of exercise and lung disease on these limiting factors.
- Describe how reaction rates with hemoglobin influence the transfer of oxygen.

From the description of Fick's law of diffusion, gas exchange between the alveoli and blood depends on a maintained diffusion gradient and favorable membrane properties. Gas exchange can become limited if:

1. There is an impediment to diffusion across the membrane (e.g., an increase in membrane thickness T or a reduction in surface area A),

OR

2. The diffusion gradient across the membrane is reduced (i.e., reduced P_1–P_2). This can occur if perfusion is too low.

Identifying whether deranged blood gases are due to diffusion or perfusion limitations can help in the diagnosis of an underlying pathological issue, so we will look at them here.

Diffusion Versus Perfusion Limitations

If a sufficient diffusion gradient exists across a membrane, then the rate of transfer of gas is primarily dependent on the properties of the membrane (see the left side of the figure 8.1). The transfer of gas in this case is referred to as a diffusion limitation.

If gas starts to accumulate on the other side of the membrane, however, the pressure gradient will dissipate and transfer rates become limited (right side of figure 8.1). This is referred to as a perfusion limitation, as it is indicative of low blood flow that is insufficient to "wash away" transferred gas, keep blood gas partial pressure low, and maintain the diffusion gradient.

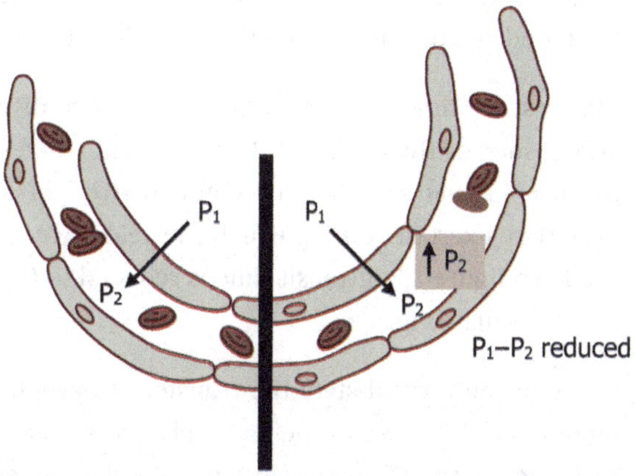

Figure 8.1: Diffusion and perfusion limitations.

We can illustrate these diffusion and perfusion limitations with the behavior of two nonphysiological gases transferring from the alveolus to the bloodstream.

Carbon monoxide is well known for its affinity for hemoglobin. When CO passes across the membrane it rapidly binds to hemoglobin and is thus removed from solution. This removal from solution maintains the pressure gradient across the membrane. So with a maintained pressure gradient the major impediment to CO transfer is diffusion across the membrane. Therefore CO transfer is referred to as diffusion limited and dependent on the properties of the membrane. (Consequently CO is used in diffusion limitation testing (DL_{CO}) in pulmonary function labs.)

Nitrous oxide, alternatively, does not bind with hemoglobin at all, so its arterial partial pressure rises rapidly as it stays in solution. So maintaining the pressure gradient is dependent on how quickly the transferred nitrous oxide is washed away by blood flow. Because of this, nitrous oxide is referred to as perfusion limited.

So while our two nonphysiological gases provide good examples of diffusion and perfusion limitations, let us see how oxygen behaves.

Figure 8.2 shows the arterial partial pressures of gases against time in the capillary—think of it as transit time; it takes 0.75 seconds for blood to pass the alveolar surface.

The blood partial pressure of CO rises very little along the capillary as it is rapidly binding to hemoglobin (Hb) (figure 8.2), the pressure gradient is maintained, and the CO is only limited by the membrane; it exhibits diffusion limitation.

The blood partial pressure of nitrous oxide, alternatively, rapidly rises (figure 8.2), and the transfer of NO becomes reliant on the rate of perfusion to maintain the gradient and gas transfer (i.e., it is perfusion limited).

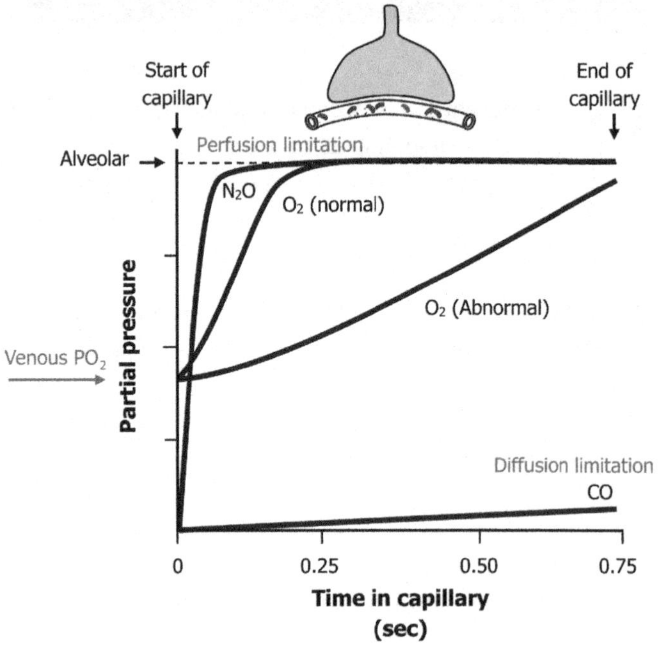

Figure 8.2: Transfer of gases from alveolus to capillary.

The results for O_2 fall much closer to the perfusion limitation (NO) line than the diffusion limitation line (figure 8.2, O_2 normal). Oxygen binds to hemoglobin so the arterial PO_2 does not rise as quickly as nitrous oxide, but the binding of O_2 is so much less than carbon monoxide it actually demonstrates more perfusion, rather than diffusion limitation.

The transfer of O_2 is also hampered by having to start off at venous partial pressures (40 mmHg), compared to our test gases that start off at zero. Consequently the initial pressure gradient is less. Despite this, the arterial partial pressure of oxygen equilibrates with alveolar pressures within 0.25 seconds (i.e., a third of the distance around the capillary). With the blood still having another 0.5 seconds in the capillary, this provides a large reserve time.

This reserve time is often eaten into in some disease states (figure 8.2, abnormal); if for example a diffusion problem arises, such as thickening of the membrane, then that extra 0.5 seconds, or last 2/3 seconds of the transit time around the alveolus, can still allow alveolar and arterial PO_2s to equilibrate. The patient may still show normal oxygen pressures until they exercise, during which the velocity of pulmonary blood flow increases and transit time is reduced; you can see from figure 8.2 if transit time is reduced to 0.5 seconds then arterial PO_2 will not equilibrate with alveolar values in the abnormal lung.

While in the normal state the transfer of oxygen is perfusion limited, in lung diseases that affect the surface area or membrane thickness of the gas exchange surface, the transfer of oxygen may become diffusion limited. Being able to measure the transfer of gas into the blood provides a valuable diagnostic tool. This is what we will look at here, not only because of its clinical pertinence, but also because it summarizes some physiological principles.

Testing the Diffusion Capacity of the Lung

The gas used to test the diffusion capacity of the lung is carbon monoxide. Why? Because as you have seen, carbon monoxide is diffusion limited, so any change in membrane characteristics will affect its movement into the bloodstream. So fundamentally, we will have the patient inhale a little carbon monoxide and hold their breath for a few seconds. During the breath-hold some CO will move into the bloodstream—the greater the disease (diffusion limitation), the more will stay in the lung. As the patient breathes out, the exhaled carbon monoxide (i.e., that not transferred) is measured. The difference between the amount inhaled and the amount returned in the exhalation is the amount that crossed into the blood. The more CO that comes back in the exhalation, the less that crossed into the blood and the worse diffusion limitation is.

Let us look at this more formally.

The transfer factor is primarily dictated by the factors within Fick's law of diffusion. Because we cannot independently measure membrane area and thickness, we lump these terms and the diffusion coefficient of the gas we are interested in into one term, the diffusing capacity of the lung, or D_L (equations below).

Equation 8.1

$$\dot{V}_{gas} = \frac{A}{T} \times D \times (P_1 - P_2)$$

↓

Equation 8.2

$$\dot{V}_{gas} = D_L \times (P_1 - P_2)$$

↓

Equation 8.3

$$D_L = \frac{\dot{V}_{CO}}{P_1 - P_2}$$

↓

Equation 8.4

$$D_L = \frac{\dot{V}_{CO}}{P_{A_{CO}}}$$

In the lab test, we are specifically looking at the transfer, or flow, of CO across the membrane, and if we rearrange this equation for transfer factor we see the transfer factor is the flow of CO divided by the pressure gradient of CO (equation 8.4). We can assume that the arterial partial pressure of CO is zero, so our equation for transfer factor ends up as the flow, or transfer, of CO across the membrane, divided by the alveolar partial pressure of CO.

But the movement of gases such as CO, and more physiologically important, oxygen, is also determined by the rate of binding with hemoglobin when it gets into the bloodstream. So our transfer factor has to contain an additional term to account for this. The rate of binding to hemoglobin is determined by two factors; first, the affinity of the gas for hemoglobin, denoted here by theta, and second, by the amount of hemoglobin present in the capillary, denoted as V_c, or capillary volume.

Equation 8.5

$$\frac{1}{D_L} = \frac{1}{D_M} + \frac{1}{\theta \times V_c}$$

So now if we rename our initial value of D_L that described the factors associated with the membrane as D_M and add our term to account for binding with hemoglobin (equation 8.5), the sum of these two gives a more complete description of transfer, or D_L. This more complete term now reflects that the transfer of gas is not solely dependent on membrane properties.

This provides a relatively simple and powerful diagnostic technique to assess disease stage and reduced function of the lung as a gas exchange organ.

Summary

So we have seen the two major factors that affect the rate of gas transfer across the lung: the rate of diffusion that is determined by the characteristics of the membrane (as described in Fick's law of diffusion), and also the rate of perfusion, which involves the rate of blood flow, volume, and binding affinity with hemoglobin. Diffusion limitation is really a description of the impediment caused by the membrane with a constant partial pressure gradient; and perfusion limitation describes whether the partial pressure gradient is being maintained.

References, Resources, and Further Reading

Text

Levitsky, Michael G. "Chapter 6: Diffusion of Gases and Interpretation of Pulmonary Function Tests." In *Pulmonary Physiology*, 9th ed. New York: McGraw Hill Education, 2018.

West, John B. "Chapter 3: Diffusion—How Gas Gets Across the Blood-Gas Barrier." In *Respiratory Physiology: The Essentials*, 9th ed. Philadelphia: Wolters Kluwer Health/Lippincott Williams and Wilkins, 2012.

Widdicombe, John G., and Andrew S. Davis. "Chapter 4." In *Respiratory Physiology*. Baltimore: University Park Press, 1983.

Figures

Figure 8.1: Diffusion and perfusion limitations. Grey, Kindred. 2022. CC BY 4.0. Added red blood cells by Lucas Helle from Noun Project. CC BY 3.0. https://archive.org/details/8.1_20220125

Figure 8.2: Transfer of gases from alveolus to capillary. Grey, Kindred. 2022. CC BY 4.0. Added red blood cells by Lucas Helle from Noun Project. CC BY 3.0. https://archive.org/details/8.2_20220125

9. Pulmonary Blood Flow

Learning objectives

- Differentiate between the pulmonary and systemic circulations with respect to: total flow rate, blood volume, vascular compliance, vascular pressures, total vascular resistance, and response to hypoxia.
- Differentiate among zones 1, 2, 3, and 4 in the lung with respect to the relationship among pulmonary vascular pressures (arterial and venous), airway pressure, and patterns of pulmonary blood flow.

The Pulmonary Vasculature

The primary role of the pulmonary circulation is to achieve gas exchange with the airspaces. Sufficient perfusion of this circulation is as essential to gas exchange as sufficient ventilation of the alveoli. Because of this role, and the fact that pulmonary vessels are exposed to airway and alveolar pressures the pulmonary circulation has some unique characteristics that are covered in this chapter.

Functional anatomy

The pulmonary circulation takes all cardiac output from the right heart via the pulmonary arteries. Thus, even at rest it has a tremendous blood flow – about 5 liters per minute, just the same as the systemic circulation. This volume enters a vast array of vessels that penetrate all the lung structure – so much so that the complete lung structure is visible from the cast of the pulmonary vasculature in figure 9.1.

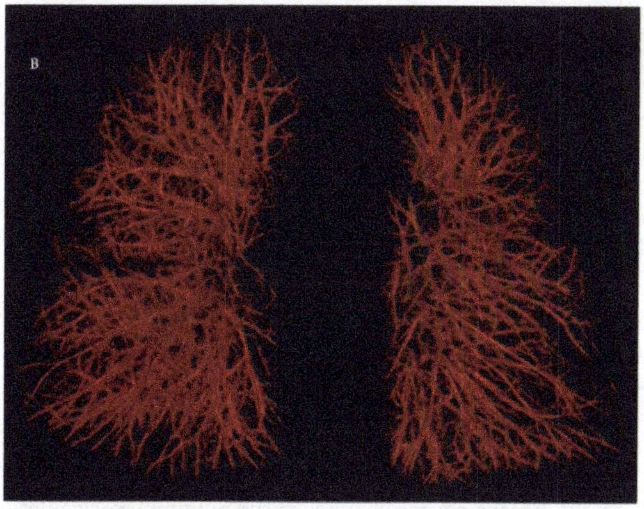

Figure 9.1: The pulmonary circulation. A latex cast of the pulmonary circulation shows the complete and vast penetration of the lung structure by the vasculature.

Main arteries follow a similar branching pattern to the bronchial tree until the terminal bronchioles are reached. This anatomical arrangement allows perfusion to follow the ventilation. Upon reaching the terminal bronchioles the vessels divide into a vast array of capillaries that wrap around the respiratory ducts and alveoli to form the respiratory zone of the lungs.

The density of the capillary beds is so great that individual capillaries can loose their distinct anatomy as can be seen in this electron micrograph where the capillaries are seen to form more sheet-like structures around where the alveoli would be. A common analogy for this is the capillaries look more like a floor of a parking garage with pillars for support but mainly open space – rather (figure 9.3) than the distinct tubes seen in other circulations.

The capillary beds converge into small veins after traveling over the alveolar surfaces, and these small veins then collect into four pulmonary veins that lead back to the left heart. This is an unusual example of veins carrying blood with arterial gas pressures.

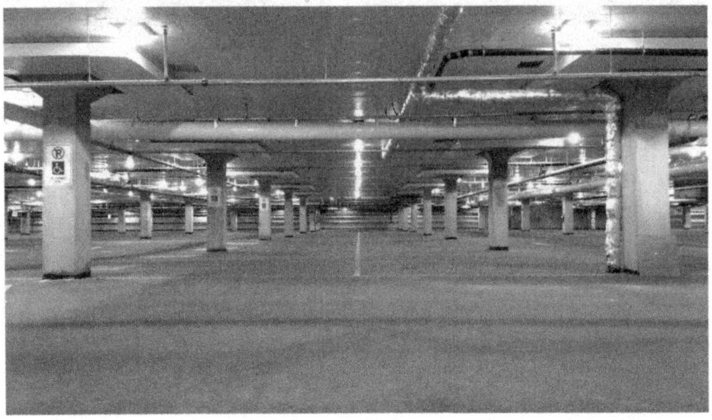

Figure 9.2: A parking garage – a bit like pulmonary capillary structure. Unlike most capillary networks that remain in distinct tubular formations, the pulmonary capillaries form something more akin to an open 'bag" of blood surrounding the alveolus with some elements of structural support, analogous to the space in this parking garage with supporting pillars.

Despite receiving the same blood volume per minute as the systemic circulation the pulmonary circulation is a low-pressure system. Systolic pressure is normally only 25 mmHg, compared to 120 in the systemic circulation, diastolic is 8, compared to 80 and mean pulmonary artery pressure is only 15. These numbers are well worth remembering.

So how can this one circulation receive so much volume (the complete cardiac output) and yet remain at such low pressure? The first reason is the vast size of the capillary beds. As figure 9.4 suggests, the much higher density of pulmonary capillary beds than that seen in the systemic circulation allows pressure to dissipate much more quickly.

The pulmonary arteries show different characteristic to their systemic counterparts as well. The walls of a pulmonary arterioles are thin compared to systemic arterioles. They also lack the smooth muscle layer seen in the systemic arteriole. In fact pulmonary arterioles look much more like systemic veins and they are often mistaken for such in biopsy or dissection. With little smooth muscle it's clear that these vessels have little role in controlling the distribution of blood flow – a vital role of their systemic counterparts. As the pulmonary circulation receives all cardiac output, all the time, such precise control isn't required.

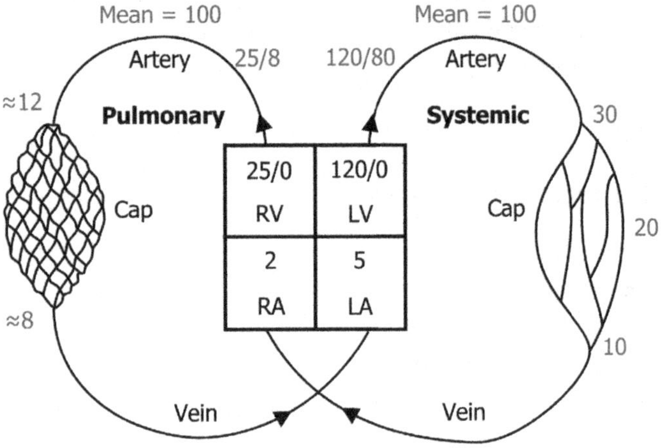

Figure 9.3: Schematic of the pulmonary and systemic circulations – compare capillary densities and pressures.

The thin walls and lack of smooth muscle also make the pulmonary arterioles highly compliant and so they behave much more like veins in their pressure response – extending when pressure increases. This gives the pulmonary arteriole system a rather unique pressure-resistance relationship that we'll look at in a moment.

This low pressure and compliant system also means that the right heart has much less work to perform to generate its output. In fact the right ventricle has about a tenth of the work of the left heart to move exactly the same blood volume. Hence the structure and work capacity of the right heart is so much smaller than the left – something worth bearing in mind if disease causes changes in the pulmonary vasculature that in turn causes the less substantial right heart to work harder and undergo hypertrophy

Pulmonary Vascular Resistance, Lung Volume, and Gravity

As we have just seen, with little smooth muscle and a compliant wall, the arterioles act more like veins. As pulmonary arterial pressure rises, the resistance of the pulmonary circulation falls, as seen in figure 9.4, and this occurs for several reasons.

Unlike systemic arterioles there is little autoregulation by the pulmonary arterioles, so the pulmonary arterioles do not actively vasoconstrict when stretched by high pressure. Instead, they passively distend, thereby reducing their resistance with increasing resistance.

A rise in pulmonary pressure not only distends vessels but initiates flow through otherwise unused, or dormant, vessels, particularly those closer to the apex of the lung (we will see why later on). With more vessels recruited, the total cross-sectional area of used vessels increases and total resistance falls.

But there are other and more complex peculiarities of the pulmonary circulation that determine its resistance...

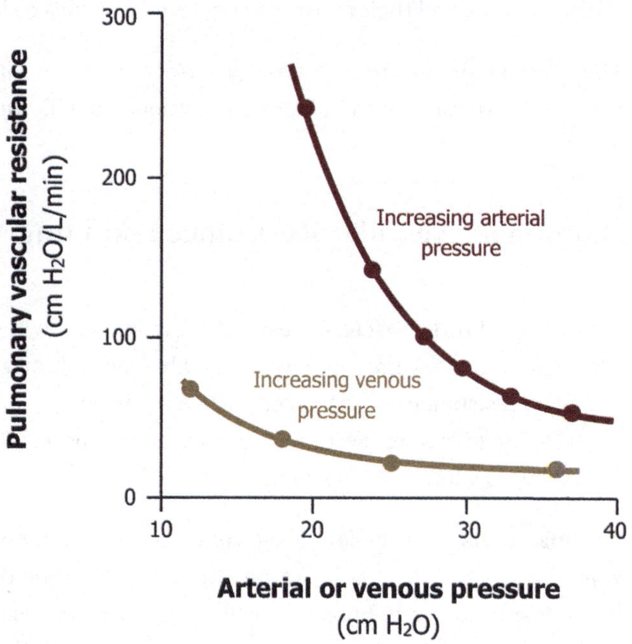

Figure 9.4: Pulmonary vascular resistance decreases as pressure increases.

Pulmonary Vascular Resistance and Radial Traction

Another unique characteristic of the pulmonary circulation is that it is exposed to the changing pressures in the airways and alveoli. It is also involved in the fiber network that generates radial traction. Consequently pulmonary vessels can be expanded or compressed in a way no other circulation is.

To explain these phenomena we have to divide the pulmonary circulation into two subdivisions, the alveolar vessels and the *extra-alveolar vessels* (figure 9.5). These two vessel types behave differently, so we will deal with them separately.

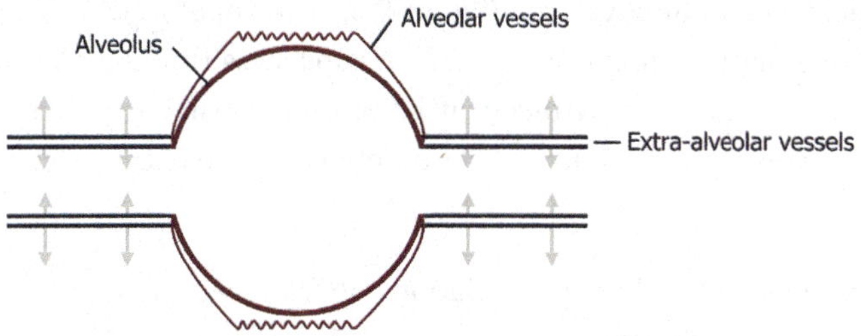

Figure 9.5: Pulmonary vessels can be categorized as alveolar or extra-alveolar.

Alveolar vessels: These are primarily the capillaries and small vessels in close contact with the alveoli. Consequently they are exposed to the alveolar pressures. First, the surface tension within the alveolus that is tending to pull the alveolus closed also pulls on the vessels between alveoli, tending to pull it open as neighboring alveoli pull inward on themselves, and play tug-of-war with the vessel walls in between, extending them and causing a decrease in vascular resistance.

Alternatively, when alveolar pressure increases (e.g., at high lung volumes), the raised alveolar pressure can compress the vessels running over its surface, causing an increase in vascular resistance.

Extra-alveolar vessels: By definition these vessels are not in contact with the alveoli, so they are not exposed to the same alveolar forces. These are exposed to the intrapleural forces, however, so as we saw airways opening during inspiration when intra-pleural pressure falls, these extra-alveolar vessels are also pulled open during inspiration by radial traction, and their resistance consequently falls as lung volume increases.

The summation of these forces (alveolar pressure, surface tension, and radial traction) means that pulmonary vasculature resistance has a complex relationship with lung volume.

Pulmonary Vascular Resistance and Lung Volume

Figure 9.6 shows vascular resistance changing with increasing lung volume. At low and high lung volumes vascular resistance is increased, while it is lower at medium lung volumes. Several forces are at play here, so let us take low lung volumes first.

Vascular resistance at low lung volumes: At low lung volumes (figure 9.6, gray zone on the left), you should know that intra-pleural pressure is less negative because the lung recoil is less. With less negative pressure to hold open the extra-alveolar vessels via radial traction, these tend to narrow and vasculature resistance becomes relatively high.

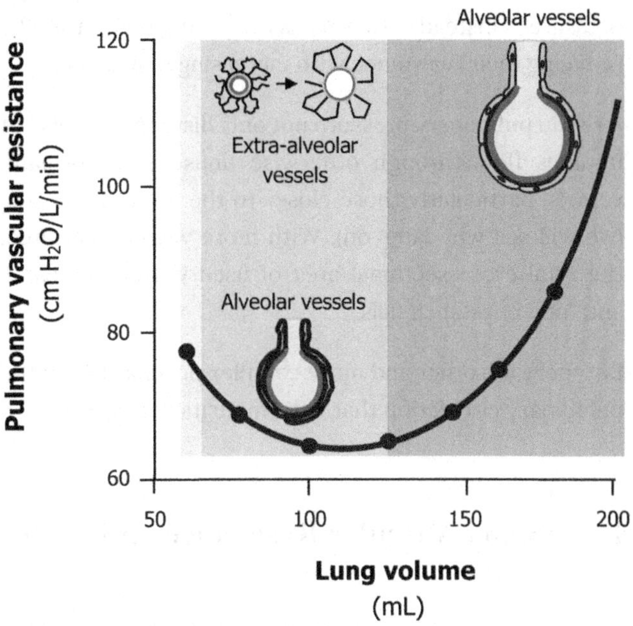

Figure 9.6: The relationship between lung volume and pulmonary vascular resistance.

Vascular resistance at medium lung volumes: As lung volume increases (figure 9.6, tan zone in the middle), the intrapleural pressure becomes more negative. Radial or parenchymal traction now begins to pull the extra-alveolar vessels open, and as they become wider, vascular resistance falls. Common sense would tell you that this effect would increase with continually larger lung volumes, and one might expect that vascular resistance would continue to decrease as lung volume increased. But this is evidently not the case.

Vascular resistance at high lung volumes: With further increases in lung volume (figure 9.6, pink zone on the right), vascular resistance rises. At high lung volumes the alveoli are enlarging, and this causes the capillaries running around them to stretch. As the capillaries stretch, they narrow—a little like how a piece of latex tubing narrows when it is stretched. This narrowing of a large number of capillaries overcomes the radial traction effect on the extra-alveolar vessels, and there is a net increase in vascular resistance.

So vascular resistance and lung volume are related with an inverted bell-shaped relationship. Now let us look at the forces that determine the distribution of blood flow across the lung structure.

Pulmonary Blood Flow and Gravity

You may recall that gravity affected the distribution of ventilation by generating the gradient of intrapleural pressures down the lung—most negative at the apex, less negative at the base.

We see a similar distribution of blood flow in the lung as well, as figure 9.7 shows with blood flow being greater at the base of the lung than it is at the apex. Again this is simply due to gravity. Gravity pushes against the blood rising from heart level, hence the base is better perfused than the apex. Because of this, gravity is responsible for matching the level of perfusion and ventilation up the lung; both are high at the bottom, and both are low at the apex. This is advantageous, as well ventilated areas need more perfusion for efficient gas exchange, and likewise there is little point in sending large amounts of pulmonary blood to poorly ventilated areas. The relationship between ventilation and perfusion (known as the V/Q ratio) that gravity establishes is not quite ideal, however, and we will see the ramifications of this less-than-perfect relationship later on. There are also other forces affecting the distribution of perfusion as well, and we can look at them now.

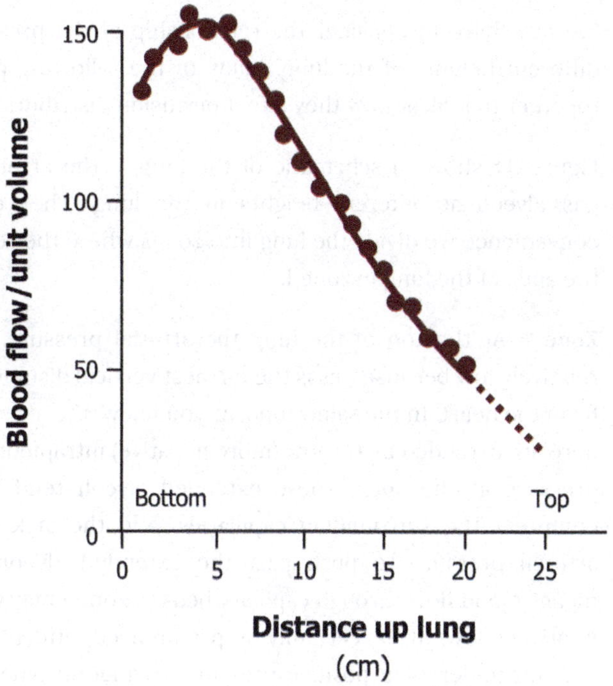

Figure 9.7: Perfusion distribution up the lung.

Zones of Perfusion

We now have to consider the relationship of the pressures in these three systems, arterial, alveolar and venous, at different heights of the lung. Many of the following principles have already been dealt with, but we can put them together to look at how they affect perfusion distribution.

Figure 9.8 shows a schematic of the lung as the arterial vessels (tan, as they carry deoxygenated blood, of course) pass alveoli at different heights in the lung. The venous system (maroon) carries oxygenated blood away. For convenience we divide the lung into zones where the relationship between these pressures changes. So we will start at the apex of the lung in zone 1.

Zone 1: At the top of the lung the arterial pressure is relatively low because this is the furthest vertical distance from the heart. In the same zone, as you know, the alveoli here are extended by the low (more negative) intrapleural pressure at the apex. These extended alveoli tend to compress the surrounding capillaries, and the lack of arterial pressure to push past the extended alveolus means blood flow through capillary beds in zone 1 may be relatively low. It is certainly a pronounced effect in patients undergoing positive pressure ventilation where alveolar pressure may exceed arterial pressure and stop blood flow at the apex altogether. This phenomenon of ventilated but underperfused alveoli is referred to as alveolar dead space, as without adequate perfusion, gas exchange is compromised.

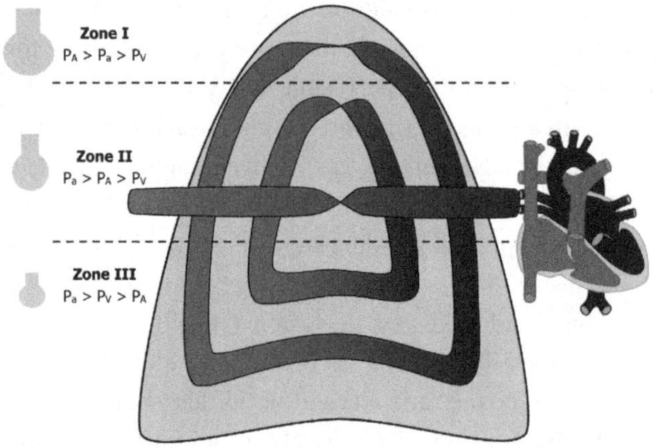

Figure 9.8: Relationships of alveolar, arterial, and venous pressures down the lung.

Zone 2: In zone 2 we are lower down the lung, and at this point arterial pressure is higher (closer proximity to the heart) and the alveoli are less extended, but venous pressure remains less than alveolar pressure. So flow in zone 2 is determined by the difference between arterial and alveolar pressures.

Zone 3: Dropping further down the lung to the base, the arterial and venous pressure have both risen as the column of fluid (blood) above them is greater at this point, and now both are above the now smaller alveolar pressure (near the base the intrapleural pressure is less negative). Consequently the flow through the capillary bed in zone 3 is determined by the arterial-venous pressure difference, just as it is in the systemic circulation.

(There can at times be a fourth zone, which appears only at low lung volumes. At low lung volumes tissue at the base of the lung can be compressed, and this compression can collapse the extra-alveolar vessels.)

Summary

So when considering flow through a systemic capillary bed we only have to think about the arterial and venous pressures, the pulmonary circulation throws us a curve ball by adding alveolar pressures into the mix that produce these perfusion zones.

Pulmonary Vasculature's Response to Hypoxia

If systemic tissue becomes hypoxic then local arterioles open to allow more blood flow and increase oxygen delivery. The opposite is true for the pulmonary circulation where the response to local hypoxia is vasoconstriction.

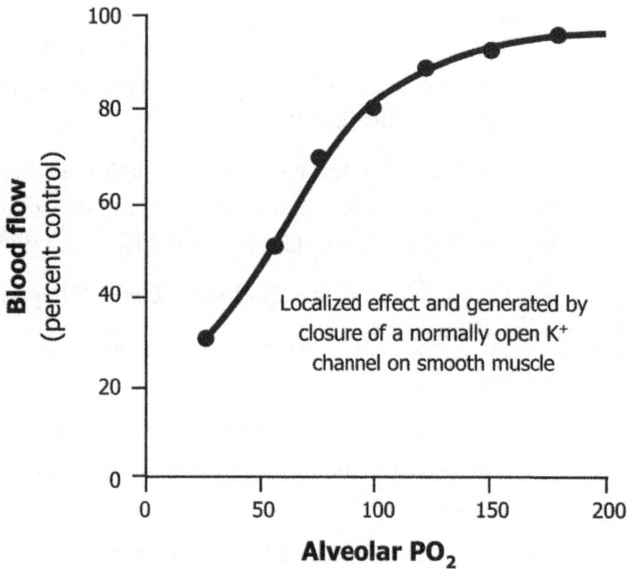

Figure 9.9: Changes in blood flow caused by vasoconstriction in response to pulmonary hypoxia.

First, remember that the bronchial circulation provides oxygen and nutrients to the pulmonary itself, and this behaves as all other systemic circulations. But the pulmonary circulation is for gas exchange. So if an area of the lung has become hypoxic (i.e., has a low oxygen partial pressure), this is indicative of that area having insufficient ventilation.

If there is little ventilation going to that area then there is little point sending perfusion to it. So the little smooth muscle there is in the pulmonary vasculature contracts to constrict the vessel when hypoxia is present. The blood follows the path of least resistance and thereby goes to vessels that are open (i.e., to areas where ventilation is maintaining a higher PO_2).

Figure 9.9 shows that blood flow increases with increasing alveolar PO_2, or more pertinently it decreases with decreasing alveolar PO_2. This shunting of pulmonary blood away from unventilated (or hypoxic) areas helps maintain matching of ventilation and perfusion (or V/Q) and efficient gas exchange.

Summary

Because of its unique role in gas exchange, rather than supplying local tissue, and the pressures that are present in the lung beyond vasculature pressure, plus the different vasculature structure, the pulmonary circulation has some unusual characteristics. These produce unique blood flow patterns in response to lung volume, gravity, and the need to match ventilated areas with adequate perfusion.

References, Resources, and Further Reading

Text

Levitsky, Michael G. "Chapter 4: Blood Flow to the Lung." In *Pulmonary Physiology*, 9th ed. New York: McGraw Hill Education, 2018.

West, John B. "Chapter 4: Blood Flow and Metabolism—How the Pulmonary Circulation Removes Gas from the Lung and Alters Some Metabolites." In *Respiratory Physiology: The Essentials*, 9th ed. Philadelphia: Wolters Kluwer Health/Lippincott Williams and Wilkins, 2012.

Widdicombe, John G., and Andrew S. Davis. "Chapter 5." In *Respiratory Physiology*. Baltimore: University Park Press, 1983.

Figures

Figure 9.1: The pulmonary circulation. Image courtesy of Dr Wei Liao, Imaging Solutions, Bayer AG Engineering & Technology, Computer Vision Innovation. 2020. Fair use. https://www.mdpi.com/2075-4418/10/12/1004/htm

Figure 9.2: A parking lot—a bit like pulmonary capillary structure. Leung, Enoch. 2018. CC BY-SA 2.0. https://flic.kr/p/28ci9r1

Figure 9.3: Schematic of the pulmonary and systemic circulations, comparing capillary densities and pressures. Grey, Kindred. 2022. CC BY 4.0. https://archive.org/details/9.4_20220125

Figure 9.4: Pulmonary vascular resistance decreases as pressure increases. Grey, Kindred. 2022. CC BY 4.0. https://archive.org/details/9.6_20220125

Figure 9.5: Pulmonary vessels can be categorized as alveolar or extra-alveolar. Grey, Kindred. 2022. CC BY 4.0. https://archive.org/details/9.7_20220125

Figure 9.6: The relationship between lung volume and pulmonary vascular resistance. Grey, Kindred. 2022. CC BY 4.0. https://archive.org/details/9.8_20220125

Figure 9.7: Perfusion distribution up the lung. Grey, Kindred. 2022. CC BY 4.0. https://archive.org/details/9.9_20220125

Figure 9.8: Relationships of alveolar, arterial, and venous pressures down the lung. Grey, Kindred. 2022. CC BY 4.0. https://archive.org/details/9.10_20220125

Figure 9.9: Changes in blood flow caused by vasoconstriction in response to pulmonary hypoxia. Grey, Kindred. 2022. CC BY 4.0. https://archive.org/details/9.11_20220125

10. Pulmonary Capillaries and Nonventilatory Function

Learning objectives

- Describe the factors that determine fluid movement between the pulmonary circulation and airspaces and how these may change to produce pulmonary edema.
- Describe nonventilatory roles of the pulmonary circulation.

Introduction

The gas exchange surface needs fluid on both the alveolar side and the capillary side for gases to dissolve into solution so they can be transported. Controlling the level of fluid on the internal alveolar surface is paramount and requires a balance between several forces. We will look at these forces here. We will also look at some of the nonventilatory roles of the lung. As the recipient of all cardiac output and with an architecture that provides a large surface area, the lung is well positioned to play other metabolic roles.

Pulmonary Capillaries and Fluid Exchange

Before looking at the unique situations that influence movement of fluid into and out of the capillary and alveoli, we will briefly review the usual Starling's forces that influence fluid movement between a capillary and the surrounding tissue.

First we will look at the balance of hydrostatic forces across the walls of a capillary as it travels through tissue. Being closest to the pumping heart, the hydrostatic pressure at the arterial end is relatively high, and likely much higher than the hydrostatic force in the interstitial space. This forms a hydrostatic pressure gradient that water moves down and out of the capillary into the tissue.

This exit of water from the capillary leaves behind a greater concentration of plasma proteins. This causes the colloid osmotic pressure to progressively rise down the capillary, and thus begins to establish an osmotic gradient with a tendency to drag water back into the capillary from the tissue. This, and the progressive drop in capillary hydrostatic pressure due to the fluid loss to the tissue and increasing distance from the heart, means most of the exuded fluid returns back to the capillary at the venous end down a hydrostatic and osmotic gradient.

The only other variable to consider here is the permeability of the capillary's endothelium and other membranes. Pulmonary capillaries are continuous and therefore normally leak relatively little, but exposure to toxins or inflammatory mediators can cause permeabilization of the capillary endothelium and increase outward fluid movement, just like a capillary in the systemic circulation.

Unlike the systemic capillaries, though, the pulmonary capillaries are exposed to airway and alveolar forces that can influence fluid movement.

Alveolar surface tension caused by the fluid lining of the internal alveolus wall not only drags the alveolar walls inward, but can also cause entry of fluid from the capillary and interstitium into the airspace. Excessive fluid accumulation can produce interstitial or alveolar edema, edema in the alveoli being much more serious as it interferes with gas exchange.

Nonrespiratory Functions of the Pulmonary Circulation

Because all cardiac output travels through the pulmonary circulation, it is ideally suited to host the enzymes needed to perform metabolic functions on blood components.

We will deal with only a few here as it is more effective to address each metabolic pathway in context of its function, rather than merely because of the location in which it occurs.

ACE: Perhaps the lung's most well-known metabolic role is to host the angiotensin-converting enzyme (or ACE). This enzyme is responsible for converting angiotensin I (released during periods of hypotension) to angiotensin II, a powerful vasoconstrictor that helps raise blood pressure. The same enzyme also inactivates 80 percent of circulating bradykinin (a potent vasodilator).

Serotonin: Other circulating substances that are controlled by the lung include serotonin, as the lung is the major site for removing serotonin from the circulation. The lung stores the serotonin, rather than breaking it down, and even transfers it to platelets who use serotonin in their hemostatic role.

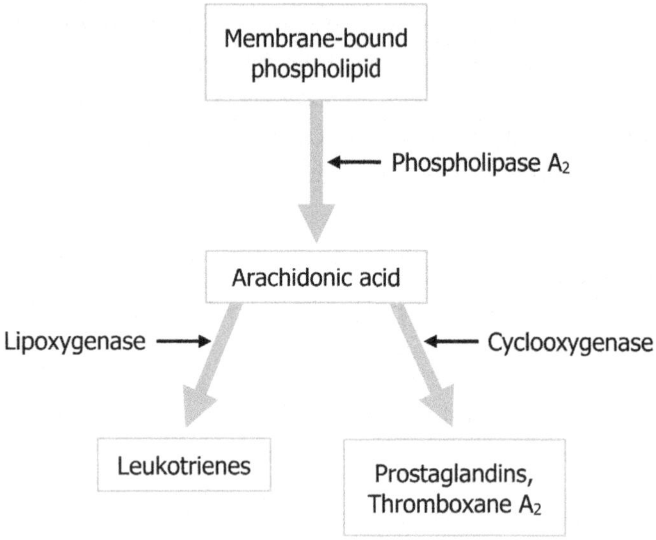

Figure 10.1: Pulmonary metabolism of arachidonic acid. Blockade of cyclooxygenase by aspirin means more arachidonic acid is available for the production of leukotrienes, which can cause bronchoconstriction.

Arachidonic acid: The lung is also involved in the metabolism of arachidonic acid, which is worth dealing with here as well because not only are the products of this metabolism vasoactive, they can also influence airway smooth muscle and cause bronchoconstriction. In brief, arachidonic acid is produced by the action of a phospholipase on membrane-bound phospholipids. The arachidonic acid can then follow one of two pathways (figure 10.1): to produce leukotrienes, which are involved in the inflammatory response and can cause bronchoconstriction, or to produce prostaglandins and thromboxane through the action of cyclooxygenases. The relevance for us here is that these alternative pathways explain why some asthmatics are sensitive to aspirin and bronchoconstrict when they take aspirin. Aspirin inhibits cyclooxygenase and thus blocks one of these pathways. Consequently there is more substrate, arachidonic acid, available for the alternate pathway and so more leukotrienes are produced, in response to which the hypersensitive airways of the asthmatic bronchoconstrict.

Summary

So from this chapter you should be able to determine the direction of fluid movement into and out of the pulmonary capillaries given the Starling and lung forces involved, and appreciate that the lung plays other relatively small but significant metabolic roles.

References, Resources, and Further Reading

Text

Levitsky, Michael G. "Chapter 10: Nonrespiratory Functions of the Lung." In *Pulmonary Physiology*, 9th ed. New York: McGraw Hill Education, 2018.

West, John B. "Chapter 4: Blood Flow and Metabolism—How the Pulmonary Circulation Removes Gas from the Lung and Alters Some Metabolites." In *Respiratory Physiology: The Essentials*, 9th ed. Philadelphia: Wolters Kluwer Health/Lippincott Williams and Wilkins, 2012.

Figures

Figure 10.1: Pulmonary metabolism of arachidonic acid. Grey, Kindred. 2022. CC BY 4.0. https://archive.org/details/10.1_20220125

11. Arterial PCO2 and pH

Learning objectives

- Describe the influence of arterial CO_2 on arterial pH.

It is often assumed that the pulmonary system's most immediate role is to maintain arterial oxygen, but this is not the case. The primary homeostatic role of the lung is to maintain a constant arterial PCO_2, and the control of breathing in humans is much more directed at this than the maintenance of arterial oxygen.

The reason control of arterial CO_2 is so critical is that it influences arterial pH. Too much CO_2 in the blood and acidosis arises, while too little raises pH to produce an alkalosis. Any deviation from a set point pH of around 7.4 can be highly dangerous as changes in pH rapidly generate changes in protein shape and function. As enzymes, membrane transporters, channels, and more start to lose function, then cellular and systemic function rapidly deteriorates. With its high metabolic rate and critical need to maintain control over its membrane potential, the nervous system is usually the first to suffer when pH changes.

So we now need to look at the relationships between CO_2, arterial pH, and alveolar ventilation. Before starting this chapter you should be completely happy that you have an understanding of pH and what constitutes a weak or a strong acid and reversible reactions.

The Influence of CO2 on pH

Active cells produce CO_2 through their anerobic and aerobic metabolic pathways. This CO_2 rapidly combines with water in the cytoplasm or plasma to produce carbonic acid. Carbonic acid is a weak acid, meaning that some but not all of it dissociates onto a hydrogen ion and bicarbonate ion. Both these molecules are critical players in the maintenance of pH, and this equation explains why CO_2 influences arterial pH.

Equation 11.1

$$CO_2 + H_2O \Leftrightarrow H_2CO_3 \Leftrightarrow H^+ + HCO_3^-$$

It is well worth committing this equation to memory and ensuring you have a good understanding of it as it is not only crucial in pulmonary pH regulation, but you will also see this equation again in renal physiology, gastrointestinal physiology, and other systems. I would argue that this is the most important equation in physiology. But let us look at it in terms of respiratory gases and the pulmonary system.

It is critical to understand that this equation is reversible, so it really describes a balance. If CO_2 at the tissue rises, the reaction is driven to the right, and consequently the amount of hydrogen ion is increased and pH falls. Conversely, if CO_2 falls, then the reaction is driven to the left, so hydrogen ion concentration falls and pH rises. Because the lung has the ability to control the expulsion rate of CO_2 from blood, the lung also has the ability to influence pH.

Physiological Context

Let us look at the most common physiological scenario: a rise in metabolic rate causes an increase in the production of CO_2 by the tissue. This, of course, pushes our equation to the right, and more hydrogen ions are produced. Because of buffering and the way CO_2 is transported in the blood (discussed later on), the rise of PCO_2 and fall of pH in venous blood is usually minimal, but both of these factors are enough to stimulate an increase in ventilation.

This increase in ventilation (more specifically, alveolar ventilation) reduces the alveolar PCO_2. This, along with a raised level of CO_2 in the venous blood, steepens the diffusion gradient from blood to alveolus. Consequently more CO_2 is transferred to the airways and expelled. This lowers blood CO_2, driving our equation back toward the left, lowering hydrogen ion concentration and returning pH back to normal.

Because of the importance of maintaining normal CO_2 (and thereby pH), alveolar ventilation exponentially increases with decreasing pH. Put simply, the ventilation control mechanisms use negative feedback reflexes to generate the appropriate level of ventilation to keep CO_2 and pH constant. Put even more simply, CO_2 is a source of acid, and the more you breathe the more CO_2 you lose, so pH rises with increased ventilation.

Summary

So now you should be able to predict what will happen to blood pH with a change in PCO_2, and what the ventilatory response should be to maintain pH at a constant level.

These basic principles form the foundation to understanding common and serious clinical situations of metabolic and respiratory acidosis and alkalosis, and how compensation normally prevents deviation from a safe but narrow pH range.

References, Resources, and Further Reading

Text

Levitsky, Michael G. "Chapter 8: Acid-Base Balance." In *Pulmonary Physiology*, 9th ed. New York: McGraw Hill Education, 2018.

Widdicombe, John G., and Andrew S. Davis. "Chapter 6." In *Respiratory Physiology*. Baltimore: University Park Press, 1983.

12. Alkalosis and Acidosis

Learning objectives

- Describe how changing alveolar ventilation leads to changes in arterial pH.
- Use blood values to determine whether a patient is in alkalosis or acidosis, and whether or not compensation is present.

Alveolar Ventilation and Arterial pH

With the help of the buffering systems and renal function, the pulmonary system plays an important role in pH homeostasis. In this chapter we will look at how the lungs contribute to the control of pH, and how failure of the pulmonary system or control of breathing can lead to dangerous deviations in pH.

CO2 and pH

We will start by revisiting the equation dealt with in the previous chapter in the context of four different clinical scenarios.

Case #1, normal: In the normal situation an increase in tissue metabolism leads to a rise in arterial CO_2, pushing the equation to the right and causing a rise in hydrogen ion concentration and a consequent fall in pH. Both the rise in CO_2 and fall in pH stimulate breathing. This increase in alveolar ventilation leads to a fall in arterial CO_2, pushing the equation back left and lowering hydrogen ions back to normal.

Equation 12.1

$$CO_2 + H_2O \Leftrightarrow H_2CO_3 \Leftrightarrow H^+ + HCO_3^-$$

Case #2, metabolic acidosis: CO_2 is by no means the only source of hydrogen ions in the system. Most metabolic pathways result in acidic by-products, and the pulmonary, renal, and buffering systems are generally battling to raise blood and tissue pH back from their tendency to turn acidic. The rise in hydrogen ions resulting from metabolic processes is referred to as metabolic acidosis. The fall in pH stimulates an increase in respiration, which in turn causes a fall in CO_2, and the lower CO_2 drives the equation to the left, reducing the number of H^+ and thereby raising pH back to normal. Here the pulmonary system has compensated for a metabolic process, and this is referred to as respiratory compensation of metabolic acidosis. The patient may now have a normal blood pH, but the CO_2 will be low. In summary, all the pulmonary system has done is get rid of one source of hydrogen ions (carbonic acid derived from dissolved CO_2) to compensate for another source of hydrogen ions it cannot do anything about (most metabolically driven acids are nonvolatile (i.e., do not vaporize into a gas the lungs can get rid of)).

The advantage of the pulmonary system being involved in pH regulation is that it is quick—a few larger breaths and arterial PCO_2 can be dropped significantly. So the pulmonary system is adept at minute-by-minute (or breath-by-breath) regulation of pH that copes admirably with short-term changes in pH. It is worth noting here that metabolic alkalosis can be reversed by reducing or even stopping breathing, allowing CO_2 to accumulate in the arterial blood and lowering pH back to normal.

The disadvantage to using the pulmonary system for compensation is that it can only mediate its effect via CO_2. So any metabolic acids are eventually dealt with by the renal system, which, although much slower, is capable of excreting any nonvolatile metabolic acids. So through a combination of rapid pulmonary CO_2 expulsion and slower but more versatile renal function, pH is normally maintained within a tight range even in the face of large metabolic changes. The kidney also has the advantage of being able to modify bicarbonate levels, which we will see the importance of when we look at the buffering systems in a moment.

Note

It is worth noting here, especially for the chemists and biochemists among you, that although equation 12.1 is a reversible reaction, it is open at both ends—the lung being able to expel or retain CO_2 at one end and the kidneys being able to retain or expel hydrogen ions and bicarbonate at the other.

Case #3, respiratory acidosis: Given its capability to influence pH, failure of the lung to expel an appropriate amount of CO_2 can lead to deviations in pH. Let us take a case of severe lung disease, say COPD, for example. The disease has diminished the ability of the lung to expel CO_2, so arterial PCO_2 rises, pushing the equation to the right and causing a fall in pH, referred to as respiratory acidosis. This acid must be immediately buffered until kidney function can be modified to begin secreting the excess hydrogen ions and even produce more bicarbonate to replenish the buffering system, a process referred to as metabolic compensation of respiratory acidosis.

Case #4, respiratory alkalosis: Likewise, if ventilation is inappropriately high with respect to CO_2 production, such as during a period of hyperventilation, then too much CO_2 will be lost and pH will fall. The alkalosis must be immediately buffered to avoid deleterious effects. Over the longer term the kidney can lower the raised pH by reabsorbing hydrogen ions and even excreting bicarbonate buffer—again this is termed metabolic compensation—but this time for an alkalosis caused by an inappropriate respiratory response.

Physiological Buffers

Although the lung's ability to expel CO_2 and the kidney's ability to excrete or absorb hydrogen ions allow close regulation of pH, their responses alone are not sufficient to prevent immediate local changes in pH at the tissue. This is the role of the buffering systems.

Buffering systems are chemicals within tissue and the blood that have the ability to absorb either hydrogen ions and/or hydroxyl ions. Once these ions are removed from solution (albeit temporarily) then their effect on pH is diminished. We will deal with buffers in the context of acids, as this is the most common physiological situation.

If you need an analogy for the function of buffers, imagine them as a chemical mop—they soak up the hydrogen ions and stop them from making a cellular mess, but the hydrogen ions, although contained, remain in the system. It is the role of the lungs and kidneys to "rinse the mop" and get rid of the hydrogen ions from the system.

There are three major chemical buffering groups in the body:

1. the bicarbonate system,
2. the phosphate system, and
3. intra- and extracellular proteins.

We will deal with the bicarbonate system as it involves the respiratory system and is also the major extracellular buffer.

Bicarbonate buffering: A buffering system consists of a weak base capable of absorbing a strong acid and a weak acid capable of absorbing a strong base. As such, the bicarbonate system involves two components: sodium bicarbonate (a weak base) and carbonic acid (a weak acid). Let us look at how it works and put it in the context of the lungs.

First let us see how a weak acid (carbonic acid) deals with a strong base, in this example, sodium hydroxide (equation 12.2).

Buffering a strong base using a weak acid:

Equation 12.2

$$NaOH = H_2CO_3$$

Sodium hydroxide is a strong base as it rapidly dissociates into a hydroxyl ion and a sodium ion.

Equation 12.3

$$\begin{matrix} Na^+ \\ OH^- \end{matrix} + H_2CO_3$$

The hydroxyl ion is the potential threat to physiological function so must be buffered. This is achieved by the carbonic acid dissociating into a hydrogen ion and bicarbonate (a process you are familiar with).

These dissociated ions now bind to form new partnerships as water and sodium hydroxide (a weak base) (equation 12.4).

Equation 12.4

$$\begin{matrix} Na^+ \\ OH^- \end{matrix} + \begin{matrix} HCO_{3-} \\ H^+ \end{matrix} \rightarrow H_2O + NaHCO_3$$

So there are a couple of things to notice here beyond watching the ions move and form new components. First, the buffering process has taken a situation with the threat from a strong base (NaOH) and toned it down to a situation with a weak base ($NaHCO_3$); the problem has not gone away, it has just been reduced (or buffered). Second, you will see that both of the components of the bicarbonate system, carbonic acid and sodium bicarbonate, appear in the equation—we have just shifted from one to the other.

Let us look at the opposite situation to see what happens when the buffering system is faced with a strong acid. This time a strong acid (hydrochloric acid) is faced with our weak base (sodium bicarbonate) (equation 12.5).

Buffering a strong acid using a weak base:

Equation 12.5

$$HCl + NaHCO_3$$

The hydrochloric acid rapidly dissociates into a hydrogen ion and a chloride ion. The hydrogen ion now threatens physiological function and must be buffered.

Our weak base dissociates into sodium and bicarbonate ions. Again our ions recombine, this time to produce harmless sodium chloride and carbonic acid (equation 12.6).

Equation 12.6

$$\begin{matrix} H^+ \\ Cl^- \end{matrix} + \begin{matrix} HCO_{3-} \\ Na^+ \end{matrix} \rightarrow NaCl + H_2CO_3$$

Notice again we have reduced but not removed the threat as we have gone from the presence of a strong acid to a weak one. Also notice that our two components in the bicarbonate system appear in the equation, and we have switched from one to the other. This should now make you realize that these two components are part of a reversible equation, and this reversible equation, even after the addition of sodium to one end, should look rather familiar (equation 12.7).

Equation 12.7

$$CO_2 + H_2O \leftrightarrow H_2CO_3 \leftrightarrow H^+ + HCO_{3-} + Na^+ \leftrightarrow NaHCO_3$$

As CO_2 is at one end of the equation you should appreciate how alveolar ventilation can influence the bicarbonate buffering system.

Because of their critical role in maintaining blood pH, bicarbonate ions are routinely measured along with arterial blood gases. Knowing what the blood pH, arterial CO_2, and bicarbonate levels are provides a very powerful and commonly used diagnostic measure allowing us not only to determine the pH status of the patient, but also the source of the problem and whether the renal or pulmonary systems are achieving compensation. Because of its power and common use, we are going to go through some fundamentals, and I am afraid that means looking at the bane of many a medical student: the Henderson–Hasselbalch equation. For those with a background in chemistry you might skip the next section, but for the rest of us, we are going to go through this step-by-step.

The Henderson–Hasselbalch Equation

What we will see is how the balance of bicarbonate and hydrogen ions determines pH, and how both of these ions can be influenced by the kidneys and lungs to keep pH constant.

First, we will take the central and most important part of the infamous equation, discarding the more innocuous ends.

Equation 12.8

$$H_2CO_3 \leftrightarrow H^+ + HCO_{3-}$$

This central portion describes the dissociation of carbonic acid into hydrogen and bicarbonate ions. But because carbonic acid is a weak acid, this dissociation is incomplete—some carbonic acid staying whole, some dissociating into the ions. The level of dissociation is described by the dissociation constant (K'), which really is the ratio of the concentrations of dissociated components to carbonic acid (equation 12.9).

Equation 12.9

$$K' = \frac{H^+ \times HCO_3-}{H_2CO_3}$$

Because we are interested in calculating the pH, however, we are more interested in the amount of hydrogen ions, so rearranging this equation for hydrogen ion concentration we see the hydrogen ion concentration is the dissociation constant, multiplied by the ratio of carbonic acid and bicarbonate (equation 12.10).

Equation 12.10

$$H^+ = K' \times \frac{H_2CO_3}{HCO_3-}$$

This equation theoretically would allow us to now determine hydrogen concentration and therefore pH, but there are some practical problems for us, the first of which is that the instability of carbonic acid means we cannot measure its concentration. So we have to use a proxy measure. The amount of carbonic acid is determined by the amount of carbon dioxide, as can be seen in the equation that is so familiar to you—the greater the amount of CO_2, the more carbonic acid.

Equation 12.11

$$CO_2 + H_2O \leftrightarrow H_2CO_3 \leftrightarrow H^+ + HCO_3-$$

So after accounting for the dissociation constant of carbonic acid and CO_2 and water, we can simply replace carbonic acid concentration with concentration of CO_2 (equation 12.12).

Equation 12.12

$$H^+ = K' \times \frac{CO_2}{HCO_3}$$

We then bump into our next practical problem: our equation now has CO_2 concentration in it, but clinically we do not measure CO_2 as a concentration (as in mmols), but as a partial pressure. So our next and nearly final step is to convert CO_2 concentration to CO_2 partial pressure, and we do this by multiplying the partial pressure (our measured value) by the solubility coefficient of carbon dioxide, which happens to be 0.03 mmol/mmHg. Our equation thus now can be completed using our adjusted PCO_2 (equation 12.13).

Equation 12.13

$$H^+ = K' \times \frac{0.03 \times PCO_2}{HCO_3-}$$

Our equation as it is now allows us to calculate hydrogen ion concentration, but we need pH, so we have to make a conversion. Because pH is the negative logarithm of hydrogen concentration, we express everything in the negative log form. And because the negative log of the dissociation constant is referred to as pK, then we can simplify our equation one more step (equation 12.14).

Equation 12.14

$$pH = pK - log\frac{0.03 \times PCO_2}{HCO_3-}$$

To make our equation simple to use, we now get rid of the negative log, and so get the following (equation 12.15):

Equation 12.15

$$pH = pK + log\frac{HCO_3-}{0.03 \times PCO_2}$$

We know that the pK of the bicarbonate system happens to be 6.1, so substituting this into the equation we end up with the Henderson–Hasselbalch equation (equation 12.16).

Let us put this in context.

First, the equation shows that if CO_2 rises then pH falls, and because CO_2 is under the influence of alveolar ventilation, this explains how the alveolar ventilation can now control pH. It also shows that if bicarbonate increases then pH increases, and equally if bicarbonate falls then pH falls. Because the bicarbonate concentration can be modified either way by the kidneys, the equation also shows how the kidneys can modify pH (equation 12.16).

Equation 12.16

Role of kidneys (numerator) / Role of lungs (denominator)

$$pH = 6.1 + log\frac{HCO_3-}{0.03 \times PCO_2}$$

The involvement of these two major physiological systems in this equation make the bicarbonate system a very powerful buffer, particularly when considering that there is an unlimited source of CO_2 and therefore bicarbonate supplied by the metabolism.

But more importantly it shows that pH is actually determined by the ratio of bicarbonate and CO_2 and that both are equally important. This fact is critical to appreciate as it forms the basis of understanding the compensation mechanisms we dealt with earlier. This is why I put you through this derivation. So for example, if a rise in CO_2 (such as in lung disease) is accompanied by an equal rise in bicarbonate (generated by the kidney), then the ratio between the two remains the same and therefore pH remains the same. Likewise, if during a fall in CO_2 the kidneys excrete bicarbonate, then pH can be kept constant. So before we finish, let us show you that the equation actually works by plugging in some numbers.

Example #1: Let us start with normal values, a PCO_2 of 40 mmHg and a bicarbonate of 24, and plug these into the equation. This comes to 6.1 plus the log of 20, which is 6.1 plus 1.3, or 7.4 (i.e., normal arterial pH).

Equation 12.17

$$pH = 6.1 + log\frac{24}{(0.03 \times 40)} = 6.1 + log(20) = 6.1 + 1.3 = 7.4$$

Example #2: Now let us look at a case of acute lung failure that has caused a rise in arterial PCO_2, but has not persisted long enough for the kidney to respond and compensate. PCO_2 has risen to 50 mmHg, and bicarbonate has not changed. Our calculation now goes to 6.1 plus the log of 16, which is 6.1 plus 1.2, and pH has fallen to 7.3.

Equation 12.18

$$pH = 6.1 + log\frac{24}{(0.03 \times 50)} = 6.1 + log(16) = 6.1 + 1.2 = 7.3$$

We now have three numbers that can give a meaningful clinical interpretation. The low pH indicates the patient is in acidosis. The raised PCO_2 suggests that this is respiratory acidosis, and the unchanged bicarbonate suggests no metabolic compensation has taken place.

Example #3: Now let us return to our patient thirty-six hours later when we have given the kidney a chance to respond. The patient's PCO_2 remains at 50 because of the persistent lung problem, but the kidney has raised the bicarbonate to 30. Now our equation becomes 6.1 plus the log of 20, or 6.1 plus 1.3, and pH is 7.4—apparently normal.

Equation 12.19

$$pH = 6.1 + log\frac{30}{(0.03 \times 50)} = 6.1 + log(20) = 6.1 + 1.3 = 7.4$$

But when we look at all three numbers we see that the patient is far from normal: the pH is okay only because the kidneys have raised bicarbonate to match the raised CO_2 and keep the ratio the same. So we now have a respiratory acidosis with metabolic compensation.

Summary

So although it has been a long journey through this chapter you should now be able to interpret blood gas values to determine whether a patient is in acidosis or alkalosis and whether or not compensation is present. I strongly recommend writing the Henderson-Hasselbalch equation as a formula in Excel so that you can plug in CO_2 and bicarbonate values and see what happens to pH. By repeatedly interpreting blood gas values and pH, determining the status of a patient will rapidly become second nature.

13. Ventilation and Perfusion

Learning objectives

- Derive the consequences of changing V/Q (from 0 to infinity) on alveolar and arterial gas tensions.
- Describe the consequences of regional variation in V/Q across the lung from apex to base on alveolar and arterial gas tensions.
- Describe the response of the pulmonary vasculature to changes regional of ventilation.

Ventilation and Perfusion in the Normal Lung

As alluded to previously, in order for gas exchange to be efficient, each region of the lung must receive equal amounts of ventilation and pulmonary perfusion to its alveoli. If ventilation and perfusion are not matched, then gas exchange diminishes, particularly in the case of oxygen. The relationship between ventilation and perfusion is referred to as V/Q, which describes the ratio between ventilation (V) and perfusion (Q) for a particular lung region. Because V/Q is critical to gas exchange and as many pulmonary diseases cause ventilation–perfusion mismatches, it is well worth understanding the effect of changing V/Q on arterial gases, and the regional differences in V/Q across the lung and the lung's responses to maintain V/Q when it deviates from normal.

Let us start with a description of the ideal situation, where ventilation to alveoli is matched with the perfusion, then we will see how the lung does not quite achieve this.

Figure 13.1 shows venous blood approaching and passing two alveoli, becoming oxygenated, and then heading back toward the left heart. The ideal situation is that both alveoli are both ventilated and both perfuse and that the ventilation and perfusion ratio (the V/Q) to each is equal (i.e., 1). If this is the case, then gas exchange is highly efficient, blood PO_2 comes into equilibrium with alveolar PO_2, and consequently there is no alveolar–arterial PO_2 difference.

This is what we would expect if the lung were perfect, with uniform distribution of ventilation and perfusion to all regions and a V/Q of 1 in all regions.

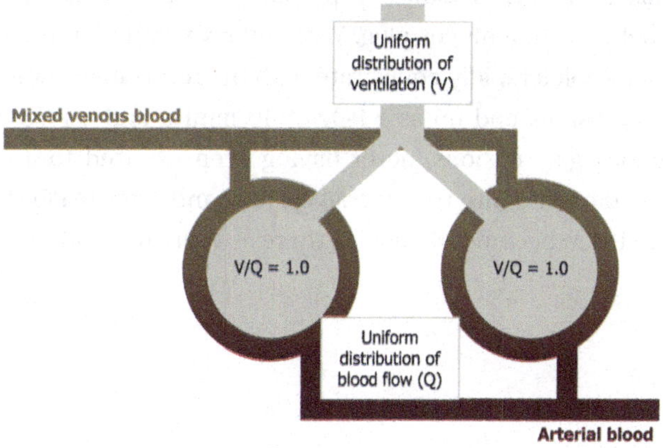

Figure 13.1: Ideal relationship of V/Q.

The lung is not a perfect organ, however, and ventilation and perfusion are not equally distributed, and the lung as a whole only achieves an average V/Q of 0.8, which is close to our ideal of 1, but not quite there. Consequently, by the time the blood has passed the alveoli and regrouped in the pulmonary veins, the PO_2 of the blood is less than alveolar. This alveolar–arterial PO_2 difference is caused by the less-than-perfect matching of V and Q across the lung; but it is not all the lung's fault, as venous blood that has been through the bronchial and a small section of the coronary circulation (and therefore is deoxygenated) is mixed into the vessels returning to the left heart, which brings down arterial saturation as well. The mixing-in of bronchial and coronary circulations and the less-than-ideal V/Q in the lung as a whole is the reason why your saturation monitors do not read 100 percent, but normal oxygen saturation is considered as 96–98 percent.

Partial Pressures and V/Q

When V and Q are matched (V/Q = 1): Atmospheric PO_2 is diluted as it descends the airways to give an alveolar PO_2 of 100 mmHg, and alveolar PCO_2 is 40 mmHg. The blood returning from the tissue has a diminished PO_2 of 40 mmHg and a raised PCO_2 of 45 mmHg. As this blood passes the alveolus, oxygen moves into the bloodstream down its pressure gradient and CO_2 moves into the alveolus down its pressure gradient. As ventilation and perfusion are matched then equilibrium is reached and the blood leaves with arterial gas tensions that are the same as alveolar tensions (figure 13.2).

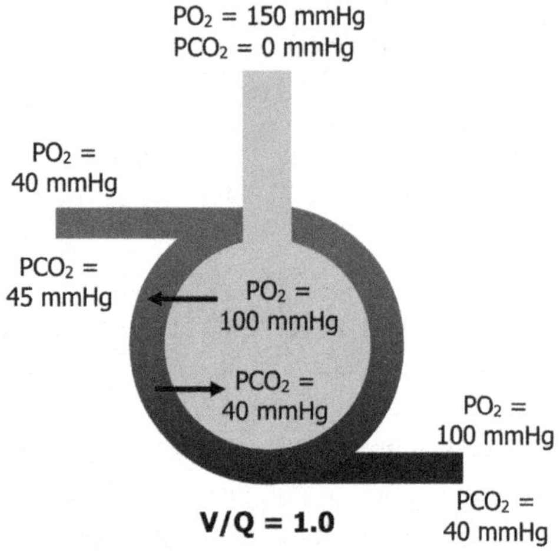

Figure 13.2: Partial pressures when V/Q = 1.

When V = 0: Now let us look at another and extreme situation, where ventilation (V) is zero so our V/Q is zero (zero divided by anything is zero).

This situation is clinically possible as airways can collapse or become blocked with a mucus plug. Without any ventilation the gas tensions inside the alveolus rapidly equilibrate with the returning venous blood, so alveolar gas tensions end up as a PO_2 of 40 mmHg and a PCO_2 of 45 mmHg. The venous gas tensions, never having been exposed to a ventilated alveolus, now circulate into the arterial system, and arterial PO_2 becomes 40 mmHg and PCO_2 becomes 45 mmHg there as well (figure 13.3).

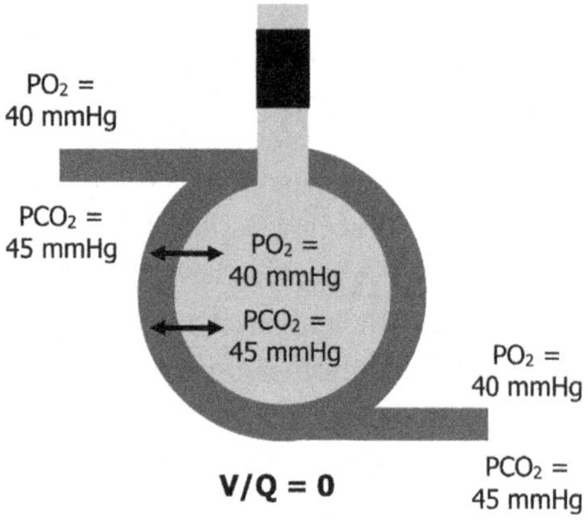

Figure 13.3: Partial pressures when V/Q = 0.

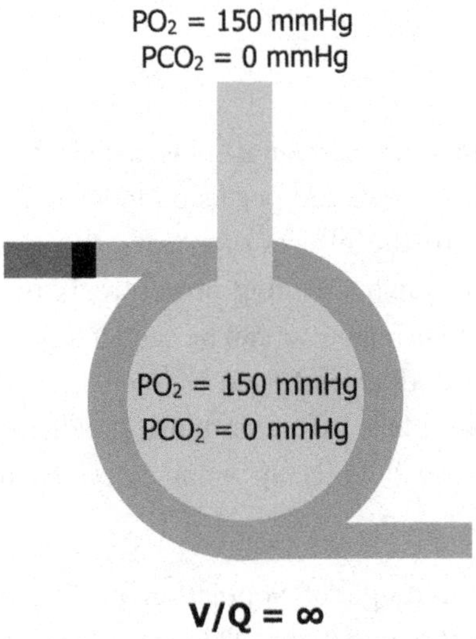

Figure 13.4: Partial pressures when V/Q is infinite.

When Q = 0: Now let us go to the other extreme, where perfusion is zero and ventilation is normal (V/Q goes to infinity). Again, this can occur in reality should a pulmonary vessel become blocked by an embolus. In this scenario V/Q becomes infinity—anything divided by zero is infinity. With no perfusion, no gas exchange occurs in this alveolus, and as it is still being ventilated then the alveolar gas tensions equilibrate with the atmosphere (figure 13.4).

So going from these extremes of V/Q as zero, passing through the ideal of V/Q of 1 to a V/Q of infinity, we get a range of alveolar gas tensions going from venous gas tensions when V/Q is zero to atmospheric gas tensions when V/Q is infinite.

This range of alveolar gas tensions is represented by the ventilation-perfusion line (figure 13.5). This graph takes a minute to come to grips with, so let us break it down. The axes of the graph show alveolar PO_2 on the X and alveolar PCO_2 on the Y. The plot shows the range of V/Q ratios we have just discussed, ranging from zero when there is perfusion but no ventilation, to infinity when there is ventilation but no perfusion. Looking at figure 13.5 more carefully will confirm our numbers. When ventilation and perfusion are present and V/Q is 1, then our alveolar PO_2 is 100 mmHg, and the alveolar PCO_2 is 40 mmHg—just as we have seen.

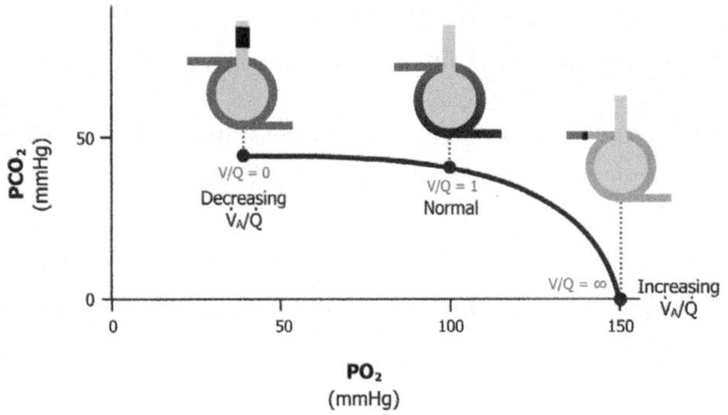

Figure 13.5: Ventilation-perfusion line.

If we stop ventilation and go to a V/Q of zero, we again see that the alveolar gas tensions become equal to venous values, with alveolar PO_2 at 40 mmHg and PCO_2 at 45 mmHg.

And finally, when we stop perfusion and V/Q becomes infinite, then alveolar PO_2 becomes 150 mmHg and PCO_2 becomes zero (i.e., equilibrates with the atmosphere).

Summary

In summary, the ventilation-perfusion line show the effect of changing V/Q on alveolar gases. Reduce V/Q toward zero and the alveolar gas tensions tend toward venous gas tensions. Increase V/Q toward infinity and the alveolar gas tensions get closer to atmospheric partial pressures.

The importance of understanding this becomes apparent when we see that V/Q changes across the structure of the lung, and if V/Q changes, then alveolar partial pressures change to.

Let us look at the distribution of V/Q across the lung and why it changes from apex to base.

Distribution of V/Q

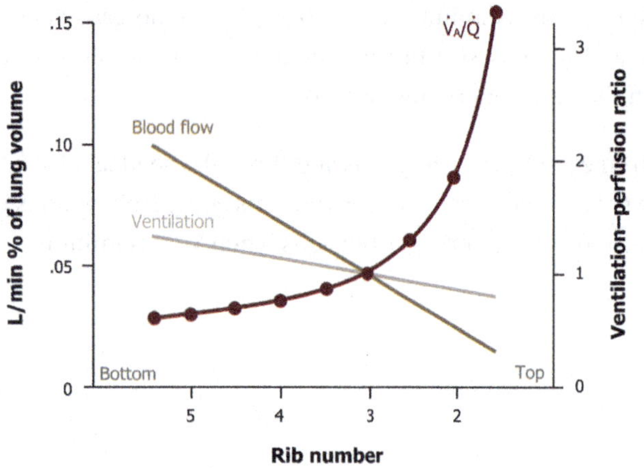

Figure 13.6: Ventilation, perfusion, and V/Q distributions.

As you should understand, ventilation increases down the lung so is greatest at the base, and perfusion follows the same pattern—all due to the effects of gravity. But the increase in ventilation down the lung structure is not equal to the increase in perfusion, as can be seen in figure 13.6. You can see here that perfusion is higher than ventilation at the base; it falls off much more rapidly as the lung is ascended, so it ends up being lower than ventilation at the apex.

This means there is a range of ventilation–perfusion ratios up the height of the lung (figure 13.6, maroon plot). At the base perfusion is higher than ventilation, so V/Q is less than 1, while toward the apex V/Q rises and becomes greater than 1. At about the level of the third rib, V/Q is perfect (yay!) as ventilation and perfusion are matched, seen here at the points the lines cross. This range of V/Q results in the previously mentioned whole lung average of 0.8.

As you should appreciate from understanding the ventilation–perfusion line, this range of V/Q across the lung results in a range of alveolar gas partial pressures across the lung. The apical alveoli, being relatively overventilated (or underperfused, whichever way you would like to think about it), have a high V/Q and consequently have partial pressures closer to atmospheric partial pressures. On the other extreme, the basal alveoli are relatively underventilated (or overperfused, your choice) and so have a low V/Q, tending toward zero; thus their partial pressures are closer to venous values (figure 13.7).

In between these two extremes is a progressive range, so what we see is that alveolar PO_2 declines down the lung while alveolar PCO_2 rises. As you might imagine, having a range of alveolar gas tensions down the lung has ramifications for gas exchange and particularly for oxygen saturation. This inequality in V/Q resulting in differences in alveolar PO_2 is substantial enough to suppress arterial oxygen saturation—and contribute to your oxygen saturation meter never reading 100 percent. Let us see why.

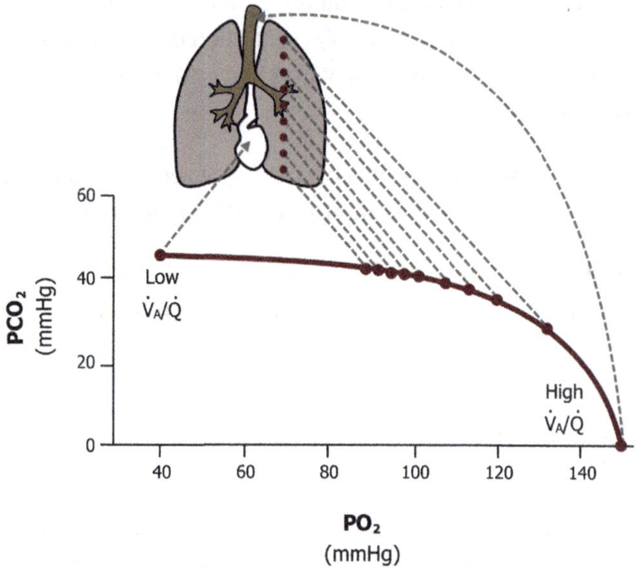

Figure 13.7: V/Q and alveolar gas distribution.

The difference in alveolar PO_2 from apex to base is as high as 40 mmHg, as is reflected in this figure. The apical alveoli have a high PO_2 (shown in figure 13.8 as 132 mmHg), primarily due to their poor perfusion and relatively high ventilation and thus high V/Q. This produces a high diffusion gradient from 132 mmHg in the apical alveoli, to 40 mmHg in the apical blood. Consequently, what blood does go to the apex becomes fully saturated before it heads back toward the left heart.

Down at the base, however, V/Q is low because of the high perfusion and relatively low ventilation. Consequently the PO_2 in basal alveoli tend toward venous values, shown in figure 13.8 as 89 mmHg. This lower alveolar PO_2 means a diminished diffusion gradient (from 89 in the alveoli to 40 mmHg in the blood), and combined with a shift down the hemoglobin saturation curve (more on this later), this means blood leaving the basal alveoli may not be completely saturated with oxygen.

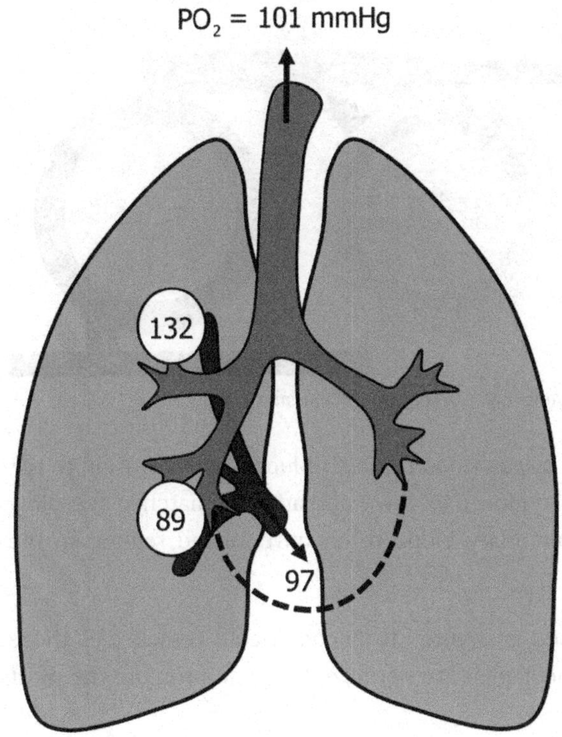

Figure 13.8: Consequences of V/Q nonuniformity on arterial PO2.

When the blood from the apex and base mix on their journey back to the left heart, the outcome is that the combined oxygen saturation is less than 100 percent, about 97 percent. It is worth making perhaps an obvious but critical point here. The blood from the apex is exposed to a substantially higher PO_2 and becomes 100 percent saturated (i.e., it cannot take on any more O_2 as it is at its full oxygen carrying capacity). There is no way that it can pick up extra to compensate for the blood coming from basal alveoli, which are not at capacity.

The same is not true for CO_2 though. Because of its high solubility, CO_2 transport does not rely on a transporter protein like hemoglobin; the transfer of CO_2 is really dependent on the diffusion gradient present. So at the apex the lower alveolar PCO_2 (slightly less than 30 mmHg looking at our V/Q line) generates a larger diffusion gradient with venous blood, and more CO_2 is transferred out the blood, meaning that it can compensate for the low diffusion gradient (perhaps only a few mmHg) that occurs between the alveoli and blood at the lung's base.

As a study exercise it may be worthwhile for you to go back to the ventilation–perfusion line and calculate the diffusion gradients for oxygen and carbon dioxide between the alveoli and venous blood at different heights in the lung. I urge you to come to grips with this concept as it is highly pertinent to respiratory disease and can explain clinical-related changes in blood gases.

The take-home message, however, is that even the normal lung is not perfect and has an average V/Q ratio of 0.8, rather than the ideal of 1, and this slight matching of ventilation and perfusion contributes to the arterial saturation being slightly less than 100 percent, but has little effect on arterial CO_2. If respiratory disease increases the mismatch, this effect on oxygen saturation can become more pronounced, but the lung has a defense mechanism for this.

Correcting V/Q Mismatches

In an attempt to maintain V/Q close to 1 and prevent V/Q mismatching, the pulmonary vasculature has an unusual response to hypoxia. While the systemic vasculature responds to local hypoxia with a vasodilation to bring more blood to the area, the pulmonary vasculature constricts in the presence of low oxygen to shunt blood away from hypoxic regions.

Let us look at a common scenario that might occur in a patient with chronic bronchitis. Figure 13.9 represents two regions of the lung. One region becomes blocked by a mucus plug, and ventilation to that region goes to zero.

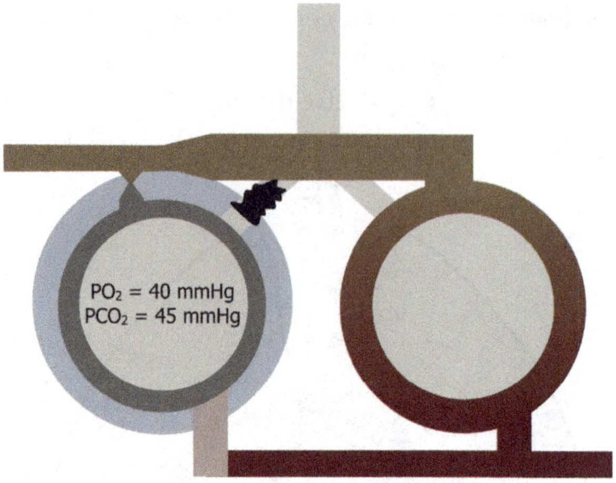

Figure 13.9: Correcting V/Q mismatches.

The alveolar partial pressures will rapidly equilibrate to venous pressures, and desaturated blood goes back to the left heart from this region while the local region around this area becomes mildly hypoxic. The pulmonary vasculature responds to the hypoxia by vasoconstricting, reducing the perfusion to the unventilated region and helping to rematch the V/Q ratio in this region (i.e., low ventilation is matched with low perfusion). In common sense terms, there is no point sending pulmonary blood to an unventilated region, so the hypoxia-driven vasoconstriction prevents this from happening.

The distensibility of the pulmonary vasculature means that the blood is shunted to unconstricted vessels (i.e., those supplying ventilated regions). Thus the lung has its own inherent mechanism to optimize V/Q and promote the most effective gas exchange possible.

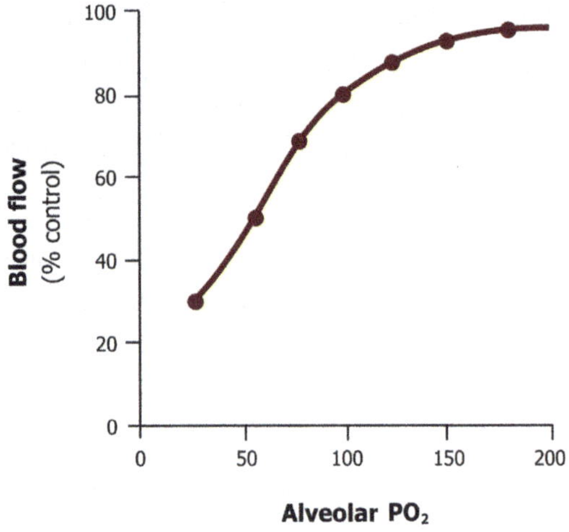

Figure 13.10: Response of pulmonary vasculature to hypoxia.

The unusual response of the pulmonary vasculature is demonstrated in figure 13.10, showing how as alveolar PO_2 falls (as occurs with a decline in alveolar ventilation) then blood flow falls—and likewise, the more oxygen in the alveolus, the more pulmonary perfusion it receives.

This effect is driven by a hypoxia-sensitive potassium channel found on the albeit sparse smooth muscle of the pulmonary arterioles. This channel is normally open and allows the exit of potassium, which in turn keeps the inside of the muscle cell polarized. When exposed to hypoxia the channel closes, and the outward potassium current stops, allowing the muscle cell's membrane potential to rise and consequently depolarize to cause a contraction.

Summary

So to summarize, the ratio of ventilation and perfusion changes across the lung, and this affects the alveolar and consequently arterial gas tensions from those regions. While the lung does not reach the ideal V/Q ratio, it is capable of shunting pulmonary blood flow away from unventilated areas to optimize gas exchange.

References, Resources, and Further Reading

Text

Levitsky, Michael G. "Chapter 5: Ventilation–Perfusion Relationships." In *Pulmonary Physiology*, 9th ed. New York: McGraw Hill Education, 2018.

West, John B. "Chapter 5: Ventilation–Perfusion Relationships—How Matching of Gas and Blood Determines Gas Exchange." In *Respiratory Physiology: The Essentials*, 9th ed. Philadelphia: Wolters Kluwer Health/ Lippincott Williams and Wilkins, 2012.

Widdicombe, John G., and Andrew S. Davis. "Chapter 7." In *Respiratory Physiology*. Baltimore: University Park Press, 1983.

Figures

Figure 13.1: Ideal relationship of V/Q. Grey, Kindred. 2022. CC BY 4.0. https://archive.org/details/13.1_20220125

Figure 13.2: Partial pressures when V/Q=1. Grey, Kindred. 2022. CC BY 4.0. https://archive.org/details/13.2_20220125

Figure 13.3: Partial pressures when V/Q=0. Grey, Kindred. 2022. CC BY 4.0. https://archive.org/details/13.3_20220125

Figure 13.4: Partial pressures when V/Q is infinite. Grey, Kindred. 2022. CC BY 4.0. https://archive.org/details/13.4_20220125

Figure 13.5: Ventilation-perfusion line. Grey, Kindred. 2022. CC BY 4.0. https://archive.org/details/13.5_20220125

Figure 13.6: Ventilation, perfusion and V/Q distributions. Grey, Kindred. 2022. CC BY 4.0. https://archive.org/details/13.6_20220125

Figure 13.7: V/Q and alveolar gas distribution. Grey, Kindred. 2022. CC BY 4.0. https://archive.org/details/13.7_20220125

Figure 13.8: Consequences of V/Q nonuniformity on arterial PO_2. Grey, Kindred. 2022. CC BY 4.0. https://archive.org/details/13.8_20220125

Figure 13.9: Correcting V/Q mismatches. Grey, Kindred. 2022. CC BY 4.0. https://archive.org/details/13.9_20220125

Figure 13.10: Response of pulmonary vasculature to hypoxia. Grey, Kindred. 2022. CC BY 4.0. https://archive.org/details/13.10_202201

14. The Alveolar Gas Equation and Alveolar–Arterial PO2 Difference

Learning objectives

- Use the alveolar gas equation to calculate the alveolar-arterial gradient of oxygen.
- Use alveolar-arterial PO_2 differences to distinguish between alveolar hypoventilation and diffusion or V/Q abnormalities.

Calculating alveolar PO2

Introduction

The difference in PO_2 in the arterial system and the alveoli of the normal lung is minimal (i.e., there is usually no substantial alveolar-arterial PO_2 difference). A fall in arterial PO_2 is indicative of a problem arising with gas exchange, but knowing whether this fall is accompanied by a growing alveolar-arterial PO_2 difference or not is a quick, cheap, and powerful diagnostic tool that can hone you in on the source of the arterial desaturation.

This chapter will describe how the alveolar-arterial PO_2 difference is calculated and what assumptions can be made from it.

Note

Before you start, a quick reminder that an uppercase A refers to alveolar and lowercase to arterial.

Calculating Alveolar PO2

Obviously to measure the alveolar-arterial PO_2 difference, we need to know both the alveolar and arterial PO_2s. The arterial PO_2 is routinely measured as part of a blood gas panel, along with arterial PCO_2. However, from your understanding of V/Q distribution across the lung, you might appreciate that the measurement of a "typical" alveolar PO_2 is difficult, and it must be calculated as an estimate of the whole lung. This is the role of the alveolar gas equation, and we will look at it now, not just because it may appear on your board exams, but primarily because of its clinical importance. As there are several forms of the equation, we will take the easy way out and use the simplest one (figure 14.1), which is accurate for the vast majority of cases you will ever see.

The alveolar gas equation estimates whole lung alveolar PO_2 as the inspired PO_2 minus the arterial PO_2 divided by the respiratory exchange ratio. For those interested in the derivation of the equation, more detailed sources are available. But here, we will just look at the factors involved and try and make this simpler to commit to memory (which I suggest you do).

First let us look at arterial PCO_2; this measurement is included in a blood gas panel so will be readily available to you. The alveolar gas equation really needs the alveolar PCO_2, but since CO_2 is so soluble then we assume that equilibration has taken place and P_aCO_2 and P_ACO_2 are the same, and we use the number we have at the bedside.

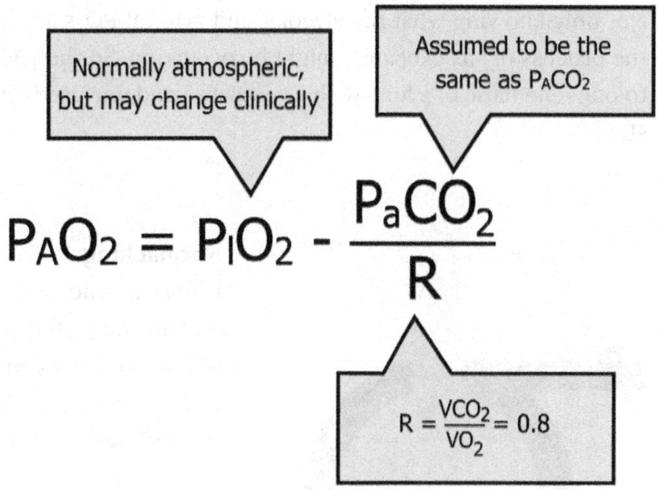

Figure 14.1: The alveolar gas equation.

Now let us look at R, or the **respiratory exchange ratio**. The respiratory exchange ratio describes how much CO_2 is produced per unit of oxygen consumed. (Perhaps you can see why we are using this in conjunction with the arterial PCO_2; we are relating CO_2 production as a proxy measurement of oxygen consumption.) When utilizing carbohydrate as a fuel (the most common situation) there are eight CO_2 molecules produced for every ten oxygen molecules burnt, so R is generally 0.8. Lastly, there is the inspired PO_2. Generally, breathing room air at sea level this will be ~150 mmHg. But it is important to note that this might change in the clinic if the patient is given oxygen therapy.

So this simple form of the alveolar gas equation really has two basic halves: the amount of oxygen taken into the alveoli (P_IO_2), and a reflection of the amount that is taken out (P_aCO_2/R) to supply metabolism.

You will find more complex and accurate forms of this equation, but for the vast majority of situations this one is perfectly adequate and is considerably easier to remember, particularly when some of the numbers we plug in are frequently the same. If we look at normal values (equation 14.1), we see that our equation gets us close to what we have learned to be a normal alveolar PO_2. Inspired PO_2 at sea level and room air is 150 mmHg, we will assume R is 0.8, and a normal arterial PCO_2 is 40 mmHg. Here is the alveolar gas equation with normal values:

Equation 14.1

$$P_AO_2 = 150 - \frac{40}{0.8} = 100$$

Now let us see the clinical use of being able to determine alveolar PO_2 and thus calculate any alveolar–arterial PO2 difference.

Alveolar–Arterial PO2 Difference and its Diagnostic Value

Not only knowing what the alveolar and arterial PO_2s are, but by how much they differ can tell us where a problem in the process of gas exchange might be occurring. So the PAO_2–PaO_2 difference has great diagnostic value. Let us return to our schematic of a lung with a ventilated and perfused lung unit and look at a few scenarios, starting with the normal state.

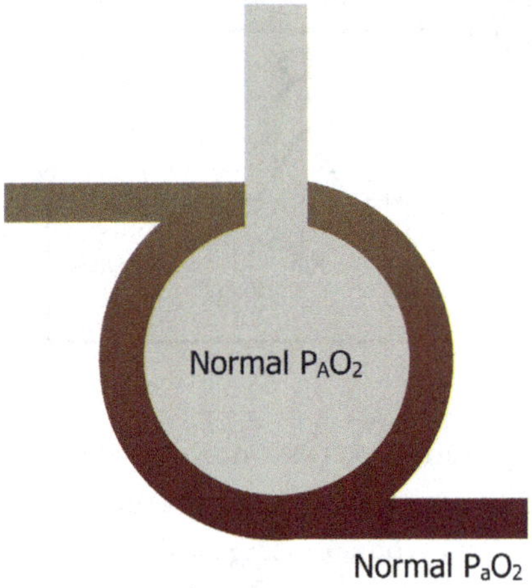

Normal $P_{A\text{-}a}O_2$

Figure 14.2: Alveolar and arterial oxygen tensions in the normal state lead to a normal alveolar-arterial PO2 difference.

Normal lung: With a well-ventilated and perfused lung (figure 14.2), alveolar PO_2 is normal, and when there are no problems with diffusion across the membrane into an adequately perfused blood vessel, arterial PO_2 is normal as well. Thus the difference between alveolar and arterial PO_2 is minimal and normal, and in reality for a young healthy person is no more than 5–10 mmHg (note, however, this difference increases with age).

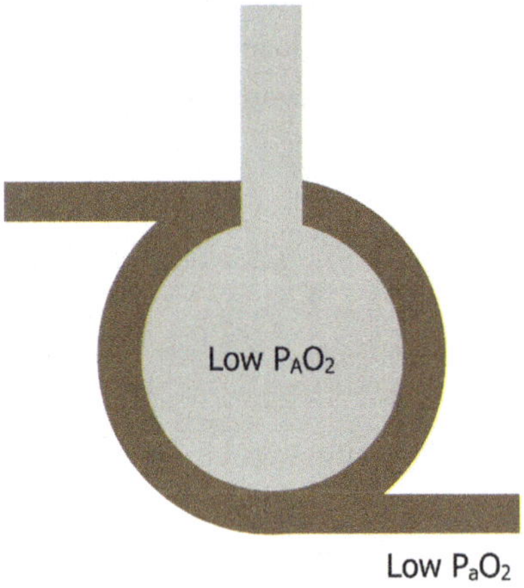

Normal $P_{A\text{-}a}O_2$

Figure 14.3: Alveolar and arterial oxygen tensions during hypoventilation result in a normal alveolar-arterial PO2 difference.

Hypoventilation: Now let us look at a case of where the alveolus is inadequately ventilated (figure 14.3): perhaps a patient has been given a high enough dose of opioid for pain relief and it has caused respiratory depression, so the patient no longer breathes enough to achieve sufficient gas exchange. This will lead to a decline in alveolar PO_2 and consequently a fall in arterial PO_2 as well. However, because the alveolar and arterial PO_2s have both decreased, then the difference between the two of them remains the same. So we see low alveolar PO_2, low arterial PO_2, but a normal A–a PO_2 difference.

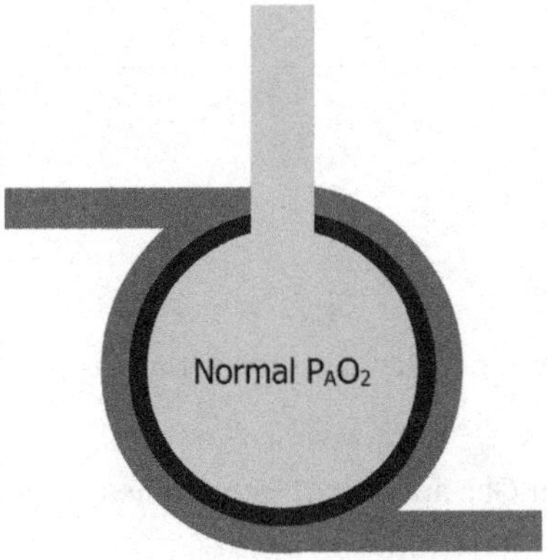

Figure 14.4: Diffusion abnormalities lead to an increased alveolar-arterial PO2 difference.

Impaired diffusion: Now let us look at a patient with a diffusion abnormality—perhaps some pathological process has caused thickening of the alveolar membranes. Here the alveolus is still adequately ventilated, so alveolar PO_2 remains high or at least the same (figure 14.4). But although blood is passing the ventilated region, the thickened membranes prevent diffusion of oxygen into the blood, and arterial PO_2 does not equilibrate and so is lower. As a consequence, the A–a difference increases. So this scenario results in a normal alveolar PO_2, a low arterial PO_2, and an increased difference between the two.

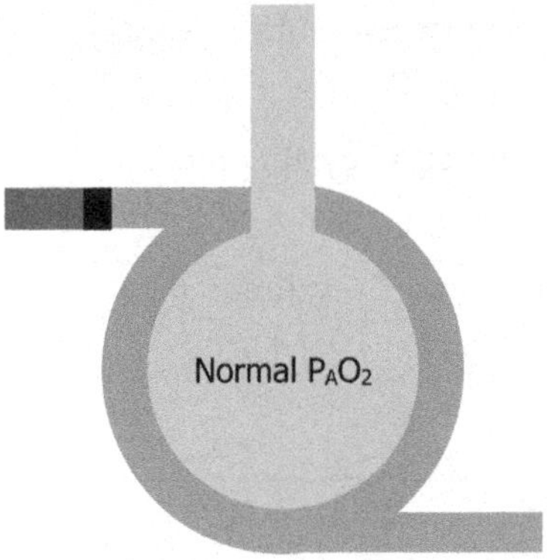

Figure 14.5: Perfusion abnormalities lead to an increased alveolar-arterial PO2 difference.

Inadequate perfusion: Now let us look at a last scenario where perfusion has been stopped, perhaps by a pulmonary embolus (figure 14.5). Ventilation still reaches the region, but there is no perfusion; this is a form of V/Q mismatch. Alveolar PO_2 remains normal because air still reaches the region, but with no perfusion and therefore no gas exchange arterial PO_2 will fall. This, again, results in an increased A–a PO_2 difference.

So what you should see from the summary in table 14.1 is that all three abnormalities cause a decrease in arterial PO_2, so all three patients are likely to present with low arterial saturations. But when blood gases are taken and the alveolar–arterial PO_2 difference is calculated, then one or more of our abnormalities could be ruled out. If there is an increased difference, you know it is not hypoventilation. If there is no increase in A–a difference, you know it is neither a diffusion problem nor a V/Q mismatch.

Summary

These examples to illustrate the point are rather specific, but generally knowing the alveolar and arterial PO_2s and calculating A–a PO_2 difference allows you to distinguish whether a decline in arterial PO_2 is due to a problem getting oxygen down into the lung, or a problem getting oxygen from lung to blood. So the alveolar equation is a simple equation, but it forms a powerful tool.

State	Effect on P_AO_2	Effect on P_aO_2	Effect on A–a PO_2
Normal	Normal	Normal	Normal (5–10 mmHg)
Hypoventilation	Decrease	Decrease	No change
Diffusion abnormality	Normal	Decrease	Increase
Lack of perfusion	Normal	Decrease	Increase

Table 14.1: Summary of Alveolar-arterial PO_2 difference.

References, Resources, and Further Reading

Text

Levitsky, Michael G. "Chapter 3: Alveolar Ventilation." In *Pulmonary Physiology*, 9th ed. New York: McGraw Hill Education, 2018.

West, John B. "Chapter 5: Ventilation–Perfusion Relationships—How Matching of Gas and Blood Determines Gas Exchange." In *Respiratory Physiology: The Essentials*, 9th ed. Philadelphia: Wolters Kluwer Health/ Lippincott Williams and Wilkins, 2012.

Figures

Figure 14.1: The alveolar gas equation. Grey, Kindred. 2022. CC BY 4.0. https://archive.org/details/14.1_20220125

Figure 14.2: Alveolar and arterial oxygen tensions in the normal state lead to a normal alveolar-arterial PO_2 difference. Grey, Kindred. 2022. CC BY 4.0. https://archive.org/details/14.2_20220125

Figure 14.3: Alveolar and arterial oxygen tensions during hypoventilation result in a normal alveolar-arterial PO_2 difference. Grey, Kindred. 2022. CC BY 4.0. https://archive.org/details/14.3_20220125

Figure 14.4: Diffusion abnormalities lead to an increased alveolar-arterial PO_2 difference. Grey, Kindred. 2022. CC BY 4.0. https://archive.org/details/14.4_20220125

Figure 14.5: Perfusion abnormalities lead to an increased alveolar-arterial PO_2 difference. Grey, Kindred. 2022. CC BY 4.0. https://archive.org/details/14.5_20220125

15. Pulmonary Shunts

Learning objectives

- Calculate the proportion of shunted blood in a right-left shunt using capillary oxygen tensions.

From understanding V/Q ratios the importance of pulmonary blood passing a ventilated surface is obvious; without sufficient blood flow, ventilated regions of the lung cannot perform gas exchange. There are occasions, however, when blood bypasses ventilated regions of the lung, or bypasses the lung altogether. When this occurs the blood in question reenters the systemic arterial circulation without having performed gas exchange. This bypassing of the ventilated lung is referred to as shunting. There are examples of blood shunting even in the healthy cardiopulmonary system, but shunts may arise or worsen with disease and cause systemic hypoxemia. Here we will look at some of the causes of shunts and how to calculate their severity.

Normal Anatomical Shunts

There are two circulatory networks that normally form shunts. The bronchial circulation, that supplies the bronchi, empties its venous blood into the pulmonary veins, thereby sending slightly deoxygenated blood back toward the left heart and into the systemic arterial system. Likewise a very small portion of the coronary venous blood is returned to the left ventricle (through the thebesian veins) and thereby bypasses the lung completely before going back in the systemic circulation.

These two wayward circulations and the imperfect V/Q matching in the lung serve to suppress arterial oxygen saturation.

Abnormal Shunts

Shunts can also be created by abnormal physiology or anatomy. There are several heart structural defects that allow blood from the right heart to enter the systemic circulation and bypass the lungs altogether; one common example is a patent foramen ovale where the incomplete atrial septum between the right and left heart allows deoxygenated venous blood to directly enter the arterial circulation, bypassing, or "shunting," past the lungs.

In pulmonary disease, areas of the lung may not receive ventilation (e.g., as airways are blocked or collapsed). Perfusion to these areas is therefore wasted as no gas exchange takes place; effectively a right-left physiological shunt has formed, and V/Q approaches zero (i.e., low V and normal Q).

Detecting Shunts

There is a quick and easy way to detect whether a shunt is contributing to a patient's low arterial PO_2 by giving a patient 100 percent O_2 to breathe. The blood passing through capillaries that are exposed to the 100 percent O_2 becomes fully saturated. However, any shunted blood never "sees" the high PO_2 and consequently stays at venous PO_2. When the two routes rejoin and the blood mixes, it remains below 100 percent (i.e., the alveolar–arterial PO_2 difference is not abolished by the 100 percent O_2, and it never can be as long as the shunt exists).

Calculating the Size of a Pulmonary Shunt

Because even a small shunt can have a large effect on arterial PO_2, it is critical to determine the size of a shunt should one be suspected. Figure 15.1 shows the lungs with blood passing through as normal (Q_C), while some bypasses the heart (Q_S) and is shunted back into the systemic circulation. The size of a shunt (Q_S) is expressed as the percentage of total blood (Q_T in figure 15.1) (i.e., Q_S/Q_T). We will look now at how this is calculated from oxygen concentration. First, let us see what we know.

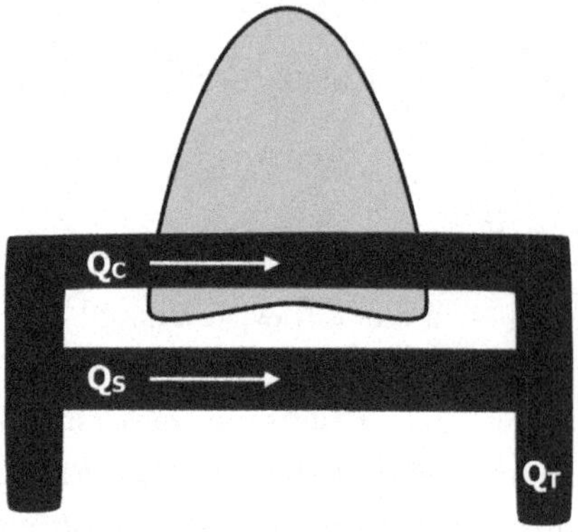

Figure 15.1: Schematic of a pulmonary shunt (anatomical or physiological) showing flow (Q) through the pulmonary capillaries (QC), flow through the shunt (QS), and total flow (QT) returning to the left heart.

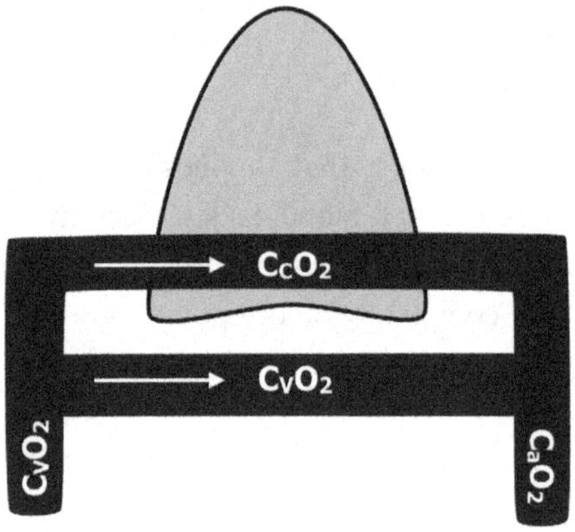

Figure 15.2: Oxygen concentrations used to calculate the size of a pulmonary shunt.

We can measure the oxygen concentration of the venous system (C_VO_2 in figure 15.2) and can assume that the shunted blood, having performed no gas exchange, will have the same oxygen concentration. We can also measure the oxygen concentration in the arterial system (C_aO_2 in figure 15.2), and if we assume that all the blood that passed through the gas exchange capillaries in the lungs equilibrated with the alveolar PO_2, we can use the alveolar gas equation to determine the capillary oxygen concentration (C_CO_2 in figure 15.2).

So know we can use these oxygen concentrations to work out the percentage of shunted blood.

Now let us combine our flow and oxygen concentration and think in terms of absolute oxygen contents in each part of our diagram. (Critical point: The absolute oxygen content is the product of the blood volume and oxygen concentration.) So now thinking of absolute oxygen contents, let us generate a first basic equation (equation 15.1) with what we know—the amount of oxygen in our flow going back to the left heart (Q_T) equals the oxygen from the pulmonary capillaries, plus that from the shunt.

Equation 15.1

$$Total\ oxygen\ content = oxygen\ from\ capillaries + oxygen\ from\ shunt$$

Let us build on that and put some values in place. The amount of oxygen arriving back in the arterial side must equal the volume of blood multiplied by the arterial oxygen concentration (Q_T x C_aO_2), as shown in figure 15.3. And we know that this amount of O_2 must be the sum of that from the capillaries, and that from the shunt.

The amount of oxygen from the shunt is calculated as shunt flow multiplied by the venous oxygen concentration (Q_S x C_VO_2), as shown in figure 15.3.

The amount of oxygen going through the pulmonary capillaries can be described as the total volume minus the shunt volume (Q_T–Q_S) multiplied by the capillary oxygen concentration (figure 15.3).

Let us put those terms into our basic equation (equation 15.2).

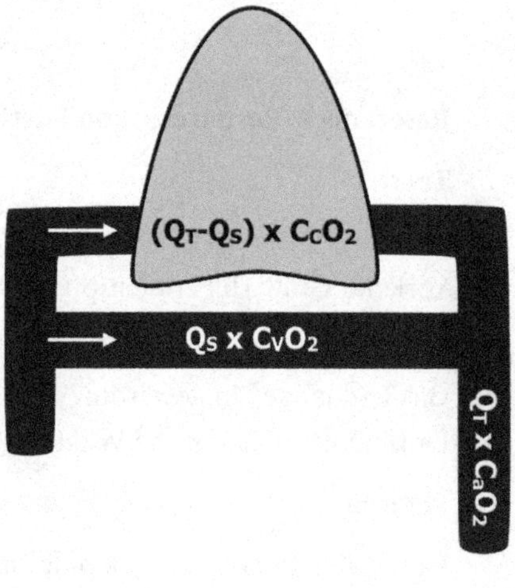

Figure 15.3: Elements of the shunt equation and where they exist physiologically.

Equation 15.2

$$\frac{Q_S}{Q_T} = \frac{C_CO_2 - C_aO_2}{C_CO_2 - C_VO_2}$$

So at this point we might panic, thinking that we have no measure of flow (Q) for any of these variables, that we only have oxygen concentrations from our blood gases and alveolar gas equation. But panic not. Through the magic of mathematics we can rearrange this equation (15.2) to eliminate our flows (Qs) and be left with an equation that meets our objective of Q_S/Q_T.

The shunt equation (equation 15.3) describes the proportion of total perfusion that is passing through the shunt. This is the equation worth remembering: the portion of blood going through the shunt is the difference between the capillary and arterial O_2 concentrations, divided by the difference between the capillary and venous oxygen concentrations.

Equation 15.3

$$Q_T \times C_aO_2 = [(Q_T - Q_S) \times C_CO_2] + [Q_S \times C_VO_2]$$

Let us look at an example to put this in context. We have a patient with normal lungs, but a right-left shunt is present. We find out that his arterial blood O_2 concentration is 18 mL and venous is 14. Capillary oxygen concentration is calculated to be 20 mL/100 mL. Now we plug the numbers in the equation and see that the proportion of blood going through the shunt is a third, or 33 percent.

Summary

So to recap, small pulmonary shunts exist even in the normal cardiopulmonary system, but abnormal shunts can arise from a number of different pathological causes. Although the presence of a shunt is relatively easy to detect, it is important to calculate its size, which is also a relatively easy process.

References, Resources, and Further Reading

Text

Levitsky, Michael G. "Chapter 5: Ventilation–Perfusion Relationships." In *Pulmonary Physiology*, 9th ed. New York: McGraw Hill Education, 2018.

West, John B. "Chapter 5: Ventilation–Perfusion Relationships—How Matching of Gas and Blood Determines Gas Exchange." In *Respiratory Physiology: The Essentials*, 9th ed. Philadelphia: Wolters Kluwer Health/ Lippincott Williams and Wilkins, 2012.

Figures

Figure 15.1: Schematic of a pulmonary shunt. Grey, Kindred. 2022. CC BY 4.0. https://archive.org/details/15.1_20220125

Figure 15.2: Oxygen concentrations used to calculate the size of a pulmonary shunt. Grey, Kindred. 2022. CC BY 4.0. https://archive.org/details/15.2_20220125

Figure 15.3: Elements of the shunt equation and where they exist physiologically. Grey, Kindred. 2022. CC BY 4.0. https://archive.org/details/15.3_20220125

16. Gas Transport

Learning objectives

- Describe how the affinity of hemoglobin for oxygen changes from the normal lung to metabolizing tissue and the local factors that contribute to these changes.
- Compare and contrast the following three terms: oxygen partial pressure, oxygen saturation, and oxygen content.
- Describe the three modes of transport of carbon dioxide by blood.

Oxygen Transport

Because of its relative lack of solubility, the transport of oxygen must involve a protein carrier, which is of course hemoglobin. In this chapter we will look at the characteristics of hemoglobin that make it an ideal and rather sophisticated carrier molecule, capable of not only picking up oxygen at the lungs, but just as importantly dropping it off at the tissue. Before that, let us briefly look at its structure (but leave most of the details to the biochemists).

The hemoglobin molecule consists of four polypeptide chains, two alpha and two beta (figure 16.1). These proteins comprise the "globin" part of the molecule but are not simply structural as they contain sites that are capable of receiving CO_2 and also hydrogen ions—a handy function, as you might imagine. Some anemias, such as sickle cell anemia, involve a conformational change in these proteins and diminish the molecule's gas carrying ability.

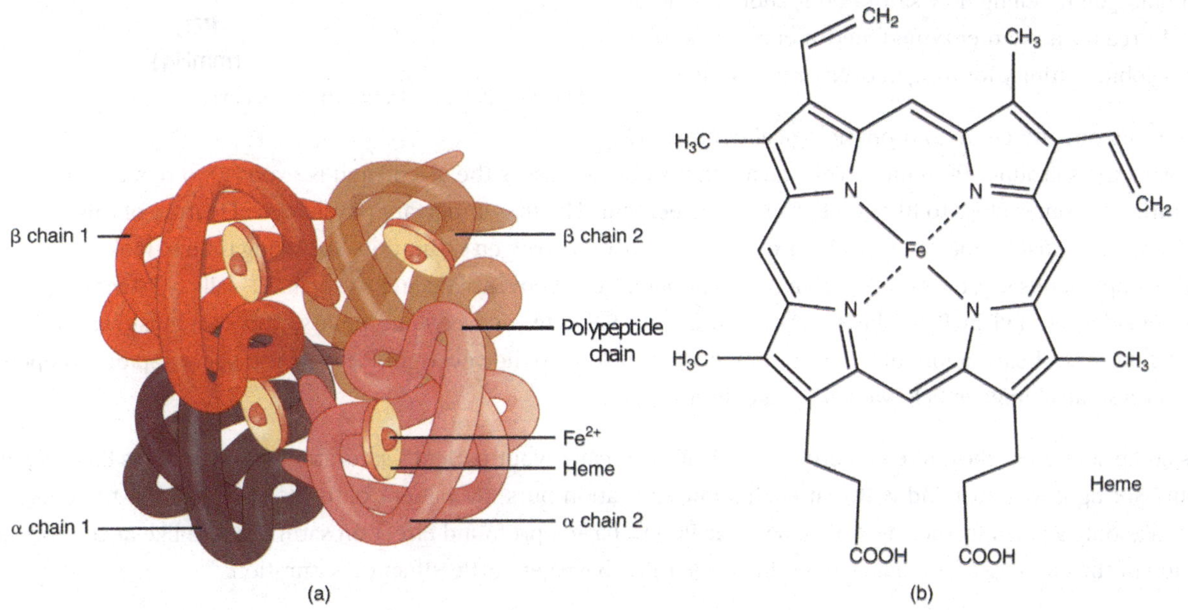

Figure 16.1: Basic structure of hemoglobin.

The heme component of hemoglobin is an iron-containing porphyrin molecule capable of binding with oxygen. Each of the four polypeptide chains contains a heme molecule, meaning that each hemoglobin molecule is capable of transporting four oxygen molecules. It is also worth noting that binding of oxygen to the heme molecule induces a conformational change that results in oxyhemoglobin having some different behaviors and indeed color to deoxyhemoglobin. We will look at some of these differences in behavior later on.

It is also worth reviewing hemoglobin's home here as well—the red blood cell (RBC). The red blood cell's classic biconcave shape provides a large surface area for gas exchange and also means that no hemoglobin molecule inside is very far from the edge of the cell, cutting down on the diffusion distance of gases. The cell is also very flexible, making it capable of squeezing through narrow and twisting capillaries so that its walls and those of the capillary may be in close contact and again diffusion distances are reduced.

Each RBC is capable of holding up to 250 million hemoglobin molecules, so consequently is capable of holding one billion oxygen molecules; as such the RBC fulfills its primary role of oxygen transport well. This oxygen transport system fails in anemias that result in either too few red blood cells or too little hemoglobin in each cell (or both). Now let us look at the behavior of hemoglobin.

The behavior of hemoglobin is best described by the oxygen saturation curve (figure 16.2), and this is one of the most important curves to understand in medicine. The curve shows the percentage of hemoglobin that has all of its heme molecules bound with oxygen (i.e., are saturated). So for example a 50 percent saturation would mean that half of the heme sites were occupied by oxygen. The curve shows percentage saturation in relation to oxygen partial pressure, and what should be immediately noticeable is that the higher the partial pressure of oxygen then the greater the saturation. But the relationship is far from linear and its shape offers several important physiological advantages. If it helps understand it, think of this curve as an instruction manual for hemoglobin, telling how saturated it should be at any PO_2. In reality it is an enzyme kinetics curve, describing hemoglobin's affinity for oxygen over a range of PO_2.

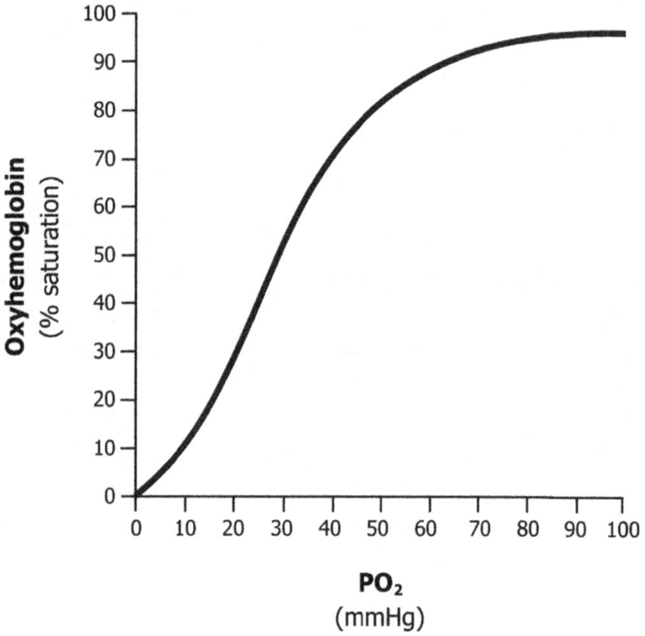

Figure 16.2: Hemoglobin saturation curve.

First let us put the curve in a physiological context. The alveolar PO_2 is around 100 mmHg. This means that as blood passes the alveoli and is exposed to this PO_2, then oxygen saturation becomes close to 100 percent, about 98 percent. The first important physiological feature of this curve is that PO_2 can fall a considerably long way before it has an impact on oxygen saturation. So, taking time to look at the numbers on the graph, let us say, for example, that a patient begins to hypoventilate and alveolar PO_2 falls to 70 mmHg; while this is a considerable fall in PO_2, the saturation will only fall a few percentage points, and PO_2 must fall to 50 before significant loss of saturation, or desaturation, occurs. Below 50, however, notice how the curve rapidly steepens, and now for a small change in PO_2, we get a large desaturation.

This steep section of the curve is therefore clinically critical. If your patient's saturation monitor reads 83 percent what should spring into your mind is it that such a low saturation puts the patient onto the steep part of the curve. It will now take only a small further decline in alveolar PO_2 to have a profound effect on saturation, unlike at the top and flat section of the curve where small changes in alveolar PO_2 have very little effect on saturation.

So what is the advantage of having such a steep curve at lower PO_2s? Let us look at the physiological situation again.

We have already said that the alveolar PO_2 of 100 results in a saturation close to 100 percent (i.e., at the lung the hemoglobin has a high affinity for oxygen and becomes fully saturated).

At the tissue, however, we want hemoglobin to lose its affinity for oxygen and release some to the metabolizing cells. At the tissue the local PO_2 is much lower, around 40, because of the oxygen consumption by the tissue. At the lower PO_2, hemoglobin's affinity for oxygen falls, and it will lose some of its oxygen to the tissue and saturation will fall. This is ideal, as now our oxygen carrier is capable of releasing oxygen where it is needed.

If tissue PO_2 falls even lower, such as when metabolic rate is high, then more oxygen will be released by hemoglobin as its affinity for oxygen declines with the lower tissue PO_2. Therefore the delivery system for oxygen is intrinsically tied to metabolic rate.

The shape of this curve makes hemoglobin a remarkable molecule—able to grab oxygen at the oxygen-providing lung, but relinquish it to oxygen-demanding tissue and relinquish more when the tissue needs more. There are other factors that fine-tune the amount of oxygen delivered to tissue to match its oxygen demand. This is summarized in figure 16.3.

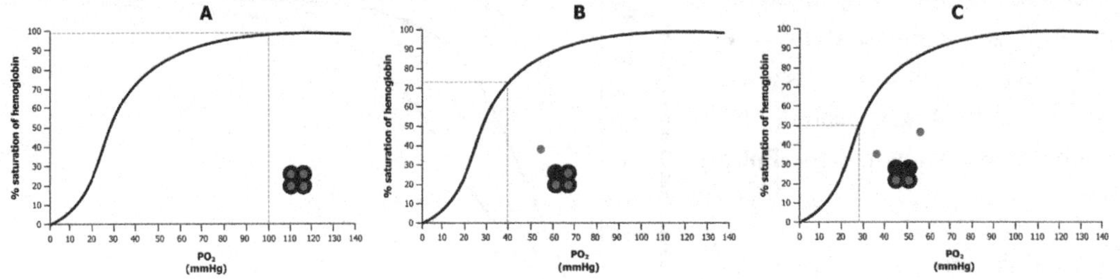

Figure 16.3: The hemoglobin saturation at the lung (A), at the tissue (B), and at very metabolically active tissue (C).

Shifts in the O_2 Saturation Curve

The metabolic rate of tissue determines its oxygen demand, with more active tissue requiring hemoglobin to relinquish more oxygen. So there are several other factors, beyond low local PO_2, that are associated with active tissue that cause hemoglobin to reduce its affinity for oxygen and therefore release it. Tissue with a high metabolic rate tends to have (1) higher temperature, (2) high PCO_2, and (3) lower pH. We can look at the effect of each of these factors on the saturation curve.

Shifts with temperature: Figure 16.4 shows the saturation curve at difference tissue temperatures. The curve we have just looked at was at 38°C. Notice that as temperature is reduced, the curve shifts to the left, but more importantly (physiologically) when temperature increases then the curve shifts to the right. Let us look at what this means in terms of hemoglobin's affinity for oxygen (follow the numbers on the graph again). As before, we will assume that our tissue PO_2 is 40 mmHg, and at normal temperatures this results in a saturation of about 70 percent.

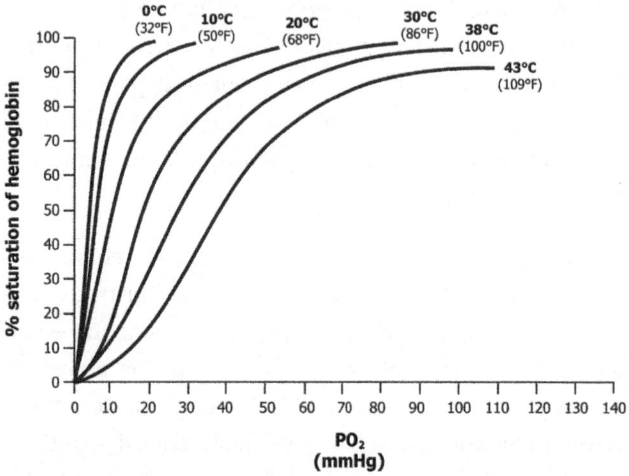

Figure 16.4: Effect of temperature on the saturation curve.

Now at the same PO_2 but a higher temperature (e.g., 43°C) the hemoglobin O_2 saturation falls to a little over 50 percent, meaning that more oxygen has been relinquished to the tissue (i.e., an increase in temperature reduces hemoglobin's affinity for oxygen).

Shifts with CO_2: We see a similar situation with a rise in PCO_2, shown in figure 16.5 with the saturation curve at different PCO_2s. At a normal arterial PCO_2 (40 mmHg) we get the same saturation curve that we saw previously. But if PCO_2 is raised, such as in the locality of highly active tissue (e.g., 80 mmHg), then the curve shifts rightward. Again this means that hemoglobin's affinity is lowered at equivalent PO_2 and more oxygen is released, resulting in a lower saturation.

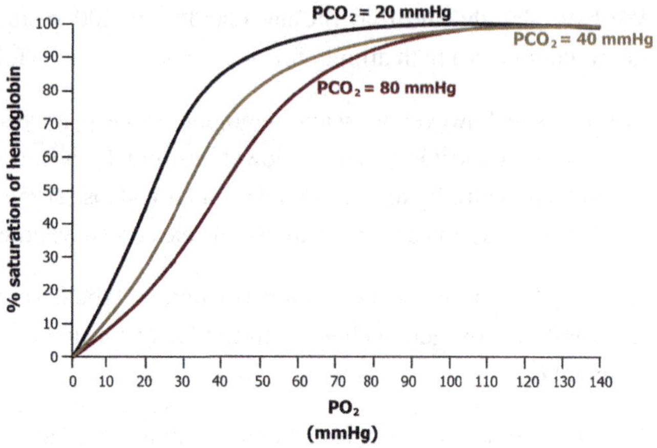

Figure 16.5: Effect of PCO2 on the saturation curve.

Shifts with pH: Finally, the same is true for changes in pH, shown in figure 16.6 with the curve at different pHs. When pH falls, as in active tissue, then the curve shifts rightward from its normal position at normal pH (7.4). Again, this result describes a lowered affinity for oxygen, so at equivalent levels of PO_2 more oxygen is released when the hemoglobin enters a low pH environment (e.g., 7.2 shown on figure 16.6). Obviously pH and PCO_2 are related, and their effect on hemoglobin binding is known as the **Bohr effect**.

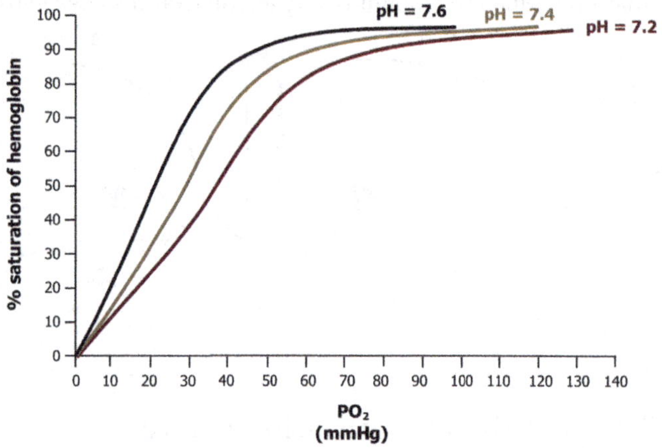

Figure 16.6: Effect of pH on the saturation curve.

One last factor that causes this rightward shift is 2,3 diphosphoglycerate, or DPG. DPG is an end product of RBC metabolism, and as it increases inside the cell it reduces hemoglobins, affinity for oxygen. Elevated DPG levels are associated with chronic hypoxia, such as experienced at altitude or more pertinently in the presence of chronic lung disease. Conversely, DPG levels are lower in stored blood, so transfused blood may have a problem giving up its oxygen.

All these factors mean that hemoglobin will deliver more oxygen to busy tissue.

Total oxygen carriage: So far we have discussed oxygen transport in terms of hemoglobin only. But despite its lack of solubility, some oxygen can dissolve into the plasma. Realistically this is a very small amount at physiological partial pressures (i.e. at an alveolar PO_2 of 100 mmHg only a fraction of a milliliter of oxygen will dissolve into the blood, as figure 16.7 shows).

Obviously this amount of oxygen is completely inadequate to support metabolism and illustrates the need for hemoglobin. But this minute amount when added to the O_2 combined to the hemoglobin makes up the total O_2 content of the blood. When calculating the oxygen content of the blood we must consider both of these compartments—hemoglobin and plasma (figure 16.8).

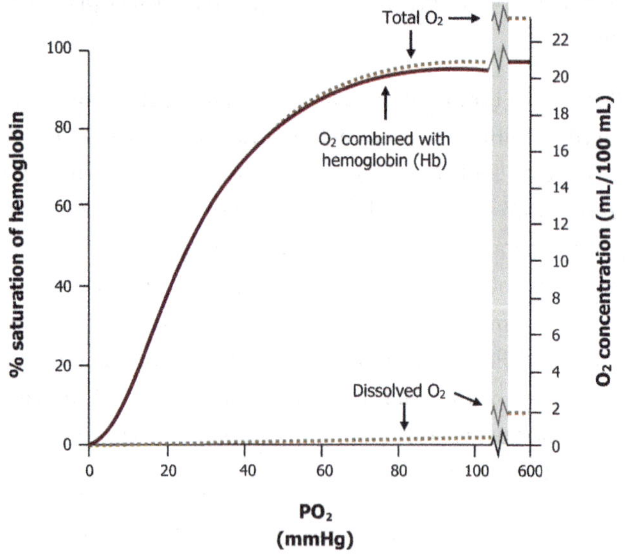

Figure 16.7: Oxygen carriage.

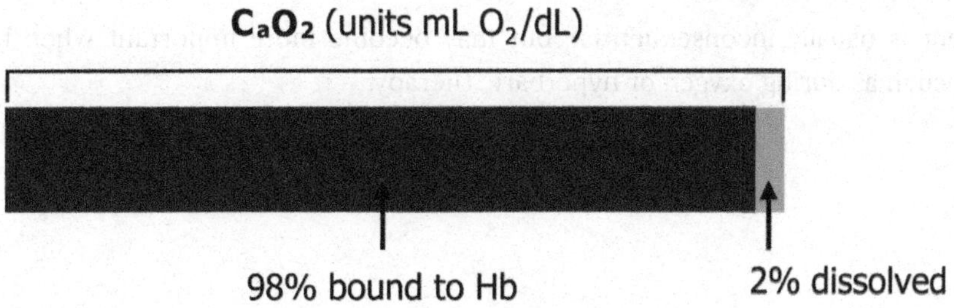

Figure 16.8: Compartment of blood oxygen content.

Calculating the O_2 Content of Blood

To calculate the arterial oxygen content (C_aO_2) let us first look at the factors affecting the majority of the O_2 (i.e., that carried by hemoglobin).

(1)
This will be determined by the amount of hemoglobin in the blood (measured in mg/dL). So let us start building the equation.

Equation 16.1

$$C_aO_2 = Hb(mg/dL)\ldots$$

(2)
Second, we must consider the oxygen carrying capacity of Hb, which is 1.34 mL O_2/gm Hb. So we multiply the amount of Hb by its carrying capacity.

Equation 16.2

$$C_aO_2 = Hb(mg/dL) \times 1.34\, O_2/gmHb\ldots$$

(3)
But that carrying capacity might not have been reached by all the Hb (i.e., the Hb may not be fully saturated). So to account for this, we multiply by the saturation (S_aO_2).

Equation 16.3

$$C_aO_2 = Hb(mg/dL) \times 1.34\, O_2/gmHb \times S_aO_2\ldots$$

(4)
So far that takes care of the O_2 associated with Hb (normally about 98 percent of the total). Now we must add the O_2 in plasma to the equation. We do this by measuring the P_aO_2 and multiplying it by a solubility coefficient (0.003 mL O_2/mmHg/dL) to convert it from a partial pressure to milliliters. Removing the units makes this long but simple equation a little easier to understand. It has two components, representing the two compartments for O_2 carriage.

Equation 16.4

$$C_aO_2 = (Hb \times 1.34 \times S_aO_2) + (P_aO_2 \times 0.003)$$

The plasma component is usually inconsequential, but may become more important when blood is exposed to an elevated alveolar PO_2, such as during oxygen or hyperbaric therapy.

Summary

So to summarize, as oxygen's lack of solubility means metabolic demands cannot be met by dissolved oxygen alone, the vast majority of oxygen is transported by hemoglobin, a molecule that is beautifully designed to pick up oxygen at the lung and release oxygen in proportion to the tissue's demand. We will see more of hemoglobin's sophistication when we address CO_2 carriage.

CO_2 Transport

Unlike oxygen, carbon dioxide is soluble enough that it does not need a protein carrier like oxygen needs hemoglobin to enter and exit plasma. However, this does not necessarily mean that CO_2 transport is simple. The complication this time is that free dissolved CO_2 forms carbonic acid, which can threaten pH homeostasis. So most CO_2 is not transported in the dissolved form. Most (approximately 70 percent) of the CO_2 that emerges from metabolizing tissue is converted to bicarbonate with the help of enzymes within red blood cells. We will look at this more closely in a moment. About 15–25 percent is transported on hemoglobin.

Transport on Hemoglobin (15–25 Percent)

Carbon dioxide can bind to the terminal amine groups of hemoglobin's polypeptide chains forming carbaminohemoglobin. It is worth noting a couple of points about this. First, CO_2 does not compete with oxygen to bind to Hb—the binding sites are completely different and hemoglobin can hold both CO_2 and O_2 at the same time. Second, deoxyhemoglobin is a better carrier of CO_2 than oxyhemoglobin is; consequently at the tissue where hemoglobin is losing its oxygen it is becoming a more efficient CO_2 transporter. This is known as the **Haldane effect**.

Transport as Dissolved CO_2 (About 7 Percent)

A little CO_2 combines with water to produce carbonic acid, the dissociated hydrogen form that must be buffered by plasma proteins, such as albumin.

Transport as Bicarbonate (About 70 Percent)

Seventy percent of the CO_2 enters red blood cells, and once inside a familiar reaction occurs (equation 16.5). The CO_2 binds with water in the cytoplasm, producing carbonic acid, which then dissociates into a hydrogen ion and a bicarbonate ion.

This reversible reaction is accelerated by the enzyme carbonic anhydrase and is driven rapidly to the right by the high concentration of CO_2 at the tissue.

The hydrogen ion produced helps shift the oxygen saturation curve to the right and so promotes further release of oxygen to the tissue. Hemoglobin then serves yet another purpose by buffering the proton with its polypeptide chains. Deoxyhemoglobin is a better proton acceptor than oxyhemoglobin, so as the hemoglobin loses its oxygen at the tissue it becomes a better pH buffer. This reduces the amount of hydrogen ion on the right side of our equation and moves the equation to the right, promoting the conversion of more CO_2.

Equation 16.5

$$CO_2 + H_2O \leftrightarrow H_2CO_3 \leftrightarrow H^+ + HCO_3-$$

High concentrations of CO_2 at the tissue push this equation right to produce bicarbonate.

The bicarbonate ion is pumped out of the cell, but without intervention this would leave the inside of the cell too positively charged as the negative charge of the bicarbonate is lost. To maintain electroneutrality the bicarbonate is exchanged for a chloride ion; this process is referred to as the chloride shift. The formation of bicarbonate at the tissue is summarized in figure 16.9.

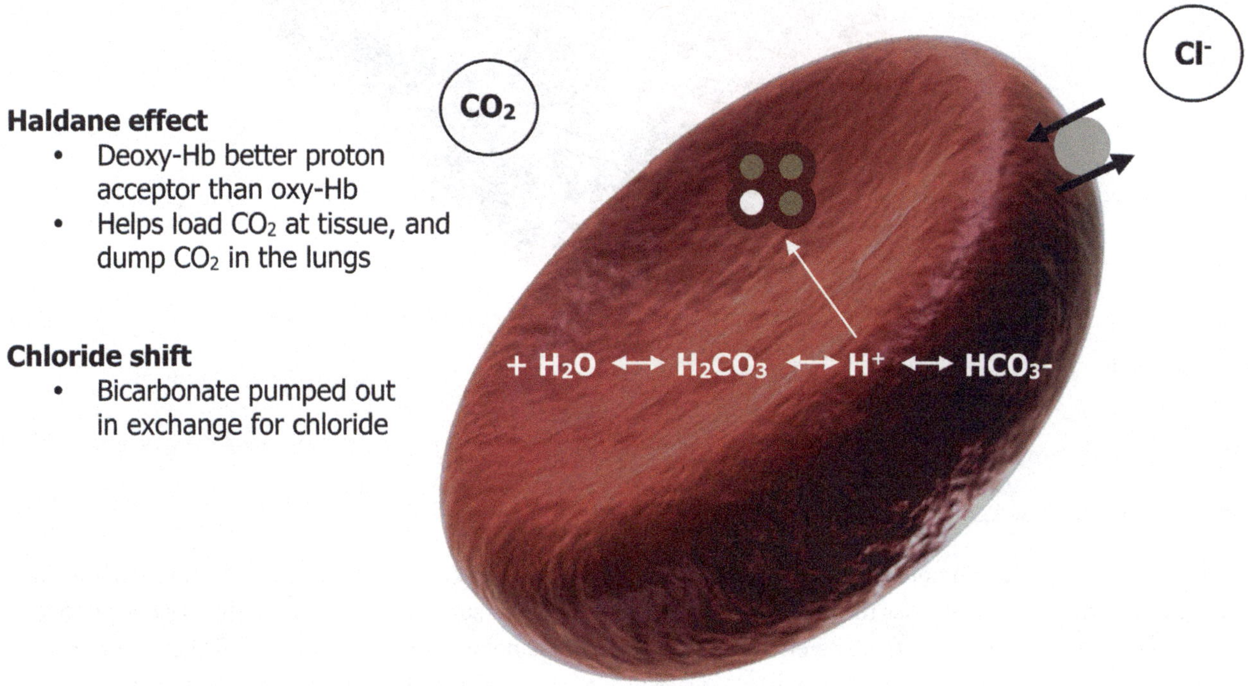

Figure 16.9: Formation of bicarbonate at the tissue.

The CO_2 now travels through the bloodstream as bicarbonate toward the lungs. At the lungs the process is basically reversed. The partial pressure of CO_2 at the lungs is low; consequently our equation is driven toward the left-hand side as CO_2 leaves toward the low alveolar PCO_2 (equation 16.6).

Equation 16.6

$$CO_2 + H_2O \leftrightarrow H_2CO_3 \leftrightarrow H^+ + HCO_3-$$

$$\leftarrow$$

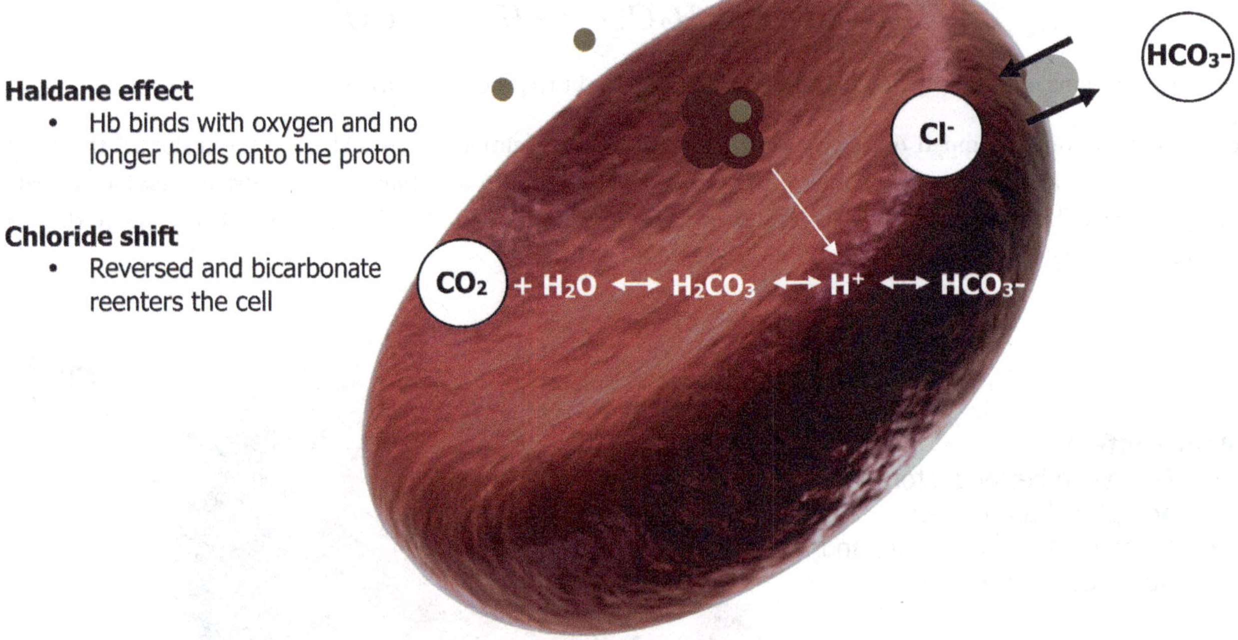

Figure 16.10: Reformation of CO2 at the lungs.

High bicarbonate and low CO_2 at the lung force the equation leftward.

The high alveolar PO_2 also promotes the leftward movement—binding of oxygen to hemoglobin makes hemoglobin a less effective proton binder so it loses the proton and raises the amount of substrate on the right-hand side and thereby promotes reformation of CO_2. The Haldane effect is also reversed—as hemoglobin gains oxygen at the lung it loses its affinity for CO_2 and releases it into the plasma. This raises plasma PCO_2 and promotes diffusion of CO_2 into the alveoli for expulsion.

Likewise the chloride shift is reversed and bicarbonate reenters the cell as chloride is pumped back out.

All these moves help promote the right-to-left direction of our now infamous equation and the re-forming of CO_2. Alveolar ventilation gets rid of the re-formed CO_2 to the atmosphere, maintaining the alveolar PCO_2 at relatively low levels and the direction of the equation right-to-left. The reformation of CO_2 at the lungs is summarized in figure 16.10.

The CO_2 "Dissociation" Curve

So, for want of a better name, we can also draw a CO_2 dissociation or saturation curve, as is shown in figure 16.11. The graph shows the CO_2 concentration in blood across a wide range of PCO_2 and shows the effect of Hb O_2 saturation on CO_2 carriage. The CO_2 dissociation curve is unlike the oxygen saturation curve and is virtually linear (i.e., the higher the PCO_2, the higher the CO_2 content of the blood); there is no plateau to the curve as we saw with O_2 transport. The ramification of this is that the lower the alveolar PCO_2, the lower the blood PCO_2, and the higher the alveolar PCO_2, the higher the blood PCO_2. It is a very simple relationship that ends with the obvious statement that the more you breathe, the lower arterial CO_2 becomes. It is worth reminding ourselves here that this is not a relationship seen with oxygen that is limited by the capacity of hemoglobin (breathing more does not necessarily result in more oxygen in the bloodstream). The other aspect to note here is the effect of hemoglobin's oxygen saturation on carbon dioxide carriage. This has clinical ramifications, so we will look at this more closely.

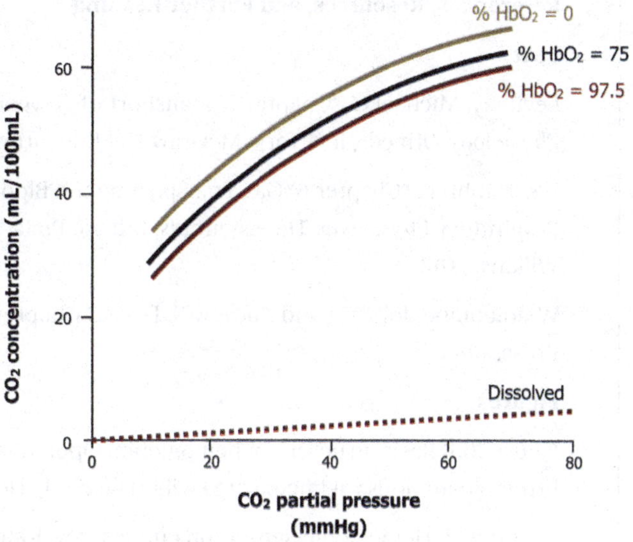

Figure 16.11: CO2 dissociation curve.

When deoxygenated, hemoglobin's structure promotes binding of CO_2 and buffering of protons by the polypeptide chains. So when O_2 saturation is zero, the CO_2 and proton carrying capability of Hb is high. As already mentioned, this means that when Hb is in its deoxygenated form at the tissue, its CO_2 carrying ability is increased.

When we get to the lung, however, the Hb is exposed to the high alveolar PO_2 and oxygen binds to the heme sites and becomes saturated; this causes a conformational change, and the CO_2 and proton carrying ability is reduced. So conveniently CO_2 release is promoted at the lung.

Summary

Although CO_2 is highly soluble, very little of it can be transported as dissolved CO_2 in plasma because of its effect on pH. The majority is converted to bicarbonate in red blood cells and transported in plasma, while about 25 percent is transported bound to hemoglobin.

References, Resources, and Further Reading

Text

Levitsky, Michael G. "Chapter 7: Transport of Oxygen and Carbon Dioxide in the Blood." In *Pulmonary Physiology*, 9th ed. New York: McGraw Hill Education, 2018.

West, John B. "Chapter 6: Gas Transport by the Blood—How Gases Are Moved to the Peripheral Tissues." In *Respiratory Physiology: The Essentials*, 9th ed. Philadelphia: Wolters Kluwer Health/Lippincott Williams and Wilkins, 2012.

Widdicombe, John G., and Andrew S. Davis. "Chapter 6." In *Respiratory Physiology*. Baltimore: University Park Press, 1983.

Figures

Figure 16.1: Basic structure of hemoglobin. OpenStax College. 2013. CC BY 3.0. https://commons.wikimedia.org/wiki/File:1904_Hemoglobin.jpg [added polypeptide chain]

Figure 16.2: Hemoglobin saturation curve. Grey, Kindred. 2022. CC BY 4.0. https://archive.org/details/16.2_20220125

Figure 16.3: The hemoglobin saturation curve. Grey, Kindred. 2022. CC BY 4.0. https://archive.org/details/15.1-needs-numbering

Figure 16.4: Effect of temperature on the saturation curve. Grey, Kindred. 2022. CC BY 4.0. https://archive.org/details/16.4_20220125

Figure 16.5: Effect of PCO_2 on the saturation curve. Grey, Kindred. 2022. CC BY 4.0. https://archive.org/details/16.5_20220125

Figure 16.6: Effect of pH on the saturation curve. Grey, Kindred. 2022. CC BY 4.0. https://archive.org/details/16.6_20220125

Figure 16.7: Oxygen carriage. Grey, Kindred. 2022. CC BY 4.0. https://archive.org/details/16.7_20220125

Figure 16.8: Compartment of blood oxygen content. Grey, Kindred. 2022. CC BY 4.0. https://archive.org/details/16.8_20220125

Figure 16.9: Formation of bicarbonate at the tissue. Grey, Kindred. 2022. CC BY-SA 3.0. Added Erythrocyte deoxy by Rogeriopfm from WikimediaCommons [added text around image]. CC BY-SA 3.0. https://archive.org/details/15.2-needs-numbering

Figure 16.10: Reformation of CO_2 at the lungs. Grey, Kindred. 2022. CC BY-SA 3.0. Added Erythrocyte deoxy by Rogeriopfm from WikimediaCommons [added text around image]. CC BY-SA 3.0. https://archive.org/details/15.3

Figure 16.11: CO_2 dissociation curve. Grey, Kindred. 2022. CC BY 4.0. https://archive.org/details/15.4_20220125

17. Control of Breathing

Learning objectives

- Identify the roles of the peripheral and central chemoreceptors in the regulation of minute ventilation.
- Describe the mechanisms that are thought to be responsible for the generation of a rhythmic pattern of breathing.
- Describe nonchemical, cortical influences on breathing.

Central Control Mechanisms

Introduction

Although control of breathing is fundamentally reflexive to maintain blood gases and pH, there are underlying complexities that, despite decades of research, are still not clear. At the foundation of ventilatory control is an underlying respiratory rhythm that can be modulated by chemoreflexes to maintain blood homeostasis, overridden by emotion or other higher brain functions, be ignored while we finish speaking a sentence (but for only so long), or be trusted to control breathing throughout the night as the rest of the brain sleeps.

In this chapter we will have a look at the regions of the nervous system that control breathing and how they interact or override each other.

The Role of the Brainstem

It has long been known that the brainstem contains critical centers for the control of breathing. These regions produce what is often referred to as the reflex drive to breathe, or brainstem drive to breathe. Despite its critical nature for survival, this involuntary motor drive that operates the respiratory muscles is barely understood.

What we will do here is summarize some basic information to create a coherent and accurate overview.

The reflex drive to breathe is a typical reflex arch, with receptors in the vasculature and lung reporting to a central controller in the brainstem that implements its effects via the respiratory muscles. What is different from most simple reflexes is that the controller is rather complex and can be thought of as a central hub that integrates inputs from multiple sources.

Many visceral sensors supplying the controller in the brainstem send their afferent signals via the glossopharyngeal and vagus nerves to the nucleus tractus solitaries, or NTS. This input station is part of an anatomically indistinct region on the dorsal surface of the medulla, called the dorsal respiratory group or DRG. The DRG connects to motor neurons that lead to the inspiratory muscles.

These DRG (figure 17.1) neurons show ramp-like bursts of activity that cause inspiratory muscle contraction to induce inspiration, then stop, allowing the inspiratory muscles to relax and passive exhalation to begin. This intermittent ramp of activity can be modulated by input from the sensors or other regions of the central nervous system, but it is not spontaneous; rather this activity is initiated by another respiratory pacemaker. It was this pacemaker that eluded physiologists for decades.

On the other side of medulla is the ventral respiratory group (figure 17.1), which has been known for a long time to contain circuits that contribute to the control of breathing within its rostral, intermediate, and caudal regions. Within the intermediate region a cluster of neurons called the pre-Bötzinger complex (figure 17.1) with apparently spontaneous activity is currently thought to be the respiratory pacemaker. The pre-bötzinger complex is likely responsible for the activity of the DRG inspiratory neurons to produce the ramping activity.

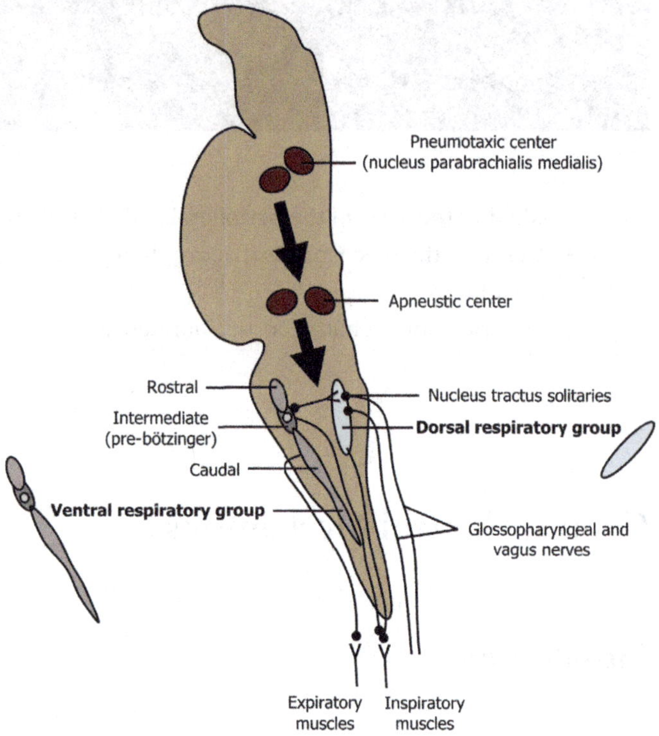

Figure 17.1: Brainstem respiratory network.

The ventral respiratory group also contains neurons with inspiratory-related activity and connections to the inspiratory motor neurons. It is better known for its expiratory neurons, however, which are capable of activating the expiratory muscles when expiration must become active rather than remain passive. During quiet resting breathing, these expiratory neurons remain dormant.

This medullary circuitry can be influenced by other brainstem centers thought to be responsible for fine-tuning the breathing rhythm.

The Apneustic center in the lower pons (figure 17.1) excites the inspiratory neurons and prolongs the ramp activity they produce; this inevitably produces a prolonged inspiratory period. Higher up in the pons is the Pneumotaxic center (figure 17.1), which acts as an off switch for inspiratory neurons; thus it regulates inspiratory volume and indirectly influences the rate of breathing, tending to increase it. This is a very basic overview of the breathing circuitry that is capable of generating inspiration and active expiration when needed. But these centers take information and direction from other neural influences, including chemoreceptors, receptors in the lung, and higher brain centers. We will look at the latter two now.

Pulmonary and Higher Brain Influences

The brainstem drive to breathe can be modulated from above and from below. The literature about whether these influences increase or decrease the drive to breathe is often confused, perhaps because of the wide range of experiments performed and the different species used. We will have a look at some of the most consistent and clinically pertinent aspects here, starting in the lung and three populations of intrapulmonary neural receptors.

Figure 17.2: Lung volume and pulmonary stretch receptor firing. The top tracing represents lung volume with two full inflations followed by a sustained inflation. In response to the increases in lung volume, pulmonary stretch receptors depolarize, producing action potentials, which are shown in the lower trace as upward spikes. The increase in action potentials with increased lung volume is seen as more densely clustered spikes. Note how the sustained inflation causes an initial high frequency of action potentials that gradually falls as the receptor adapts to the high lung volume.

Pulmonary stretch receptors are mechanoreceptors found in airway walls and smooth muscle. As their name suggests, they respond to expansion of the lung, and their afferent activity to the brainstem increases with lung volume, as figure 17.2 shows. Upon arrival at the NTS the PSR activity tends to inhibit inspiratory neurons and can stop inspiratory activity completely in other species (the **Hering–Breuer reflex**). However, their influence on the control of breathing in humans is weak, and while they might not contribute to the control of breathing in man, they likely influence respiratory sensations, such as shortness of breath.

Irritant receptors are found in the airway epithelium and are ideally placed to perform their role of detecting harmful substances entering the lungs, such as noxious gases, particulates, and even cold air. They generally have an inhibitory influence on the drive to breathe, perhaps as an attempt to limit the amount of noxious substance entering the lung. Other components to their defensive strategies are bronchoconstriction and induction of the cough reflex. Their response to inflammatory mediators also suggests they may play a role in asthma.

J-receptors, or Juxtacapillary receptors, are found at the junction of the pulmonary capillaries and alveoli. These receptors respond to increases in interstitial pressure so are likely to play a role in the response to pulmonary edema. Their effect on the drive to breathe can be regarded as excitatory as they cause an increase in breathing rate as part of the J-reflex, which includes cardiac components and is intended to prevent over-exercising and cardiopulmonary collapse. As such the J-receptors may also contribute to generating the sensation of shortness of breath.

These three pulmonary receptor groups are the three that usually appear in textbooks, perhaps because of their clinical pertinence, but perhaps because we know most about these. Others exist, and details can be found in other sources. We will now focus briefly on the influence of higher centers on breathing, and these are generally all positive (i.e., cause an increase in breathing). Cortical influences are numerous and undefined, that collectively they produce what is referred to as the wakeful drive to breath. The extent of cortical influence is best illustrated by sleep, when the higher brain is unconscious and any wakeful drive is removed. During sleep breathing is significantly reduced—enough so that arterial PCO_2 is several mmHg higher than during wakefulness. This suggests that cortical influences on breathing are enough to cause a lower P_aCO_2 than would be determined by chemoreflexes alone.

More specific influences from higher centers include emotions; anger, anxiety, sadness, happiness, and sexual arousal all influence the drive and pattern of breathing. This is perhaps best exemplified by emotionally driven sighs or the frankly bizarre activity of laughter. But the list of higher center influences does not stop there; indeed it is likely that we still yet do not know where it stops. Changes in light changes breathing, a sudden loud sound changes breathing, doing a mathematical problem changes breathing... and so on. And unfortunately for clinicians and pulmonary physiologists, the act of measuring breathing changes breathing. So it is likely that all those textbook numbers for normal respiratory rate and depth are all too high, as telling someone you are going to measure their breathing usually causes them to hyperventilate.

Breathing is also a rare incidence of being able to voluntarily control a normally reflex activity (e.g., we can willfully override reflex breathing to perform speech or a breath-hold). In fact, we have as precise control over our respiratory muscles as we have control over the muscles in our hands. Humans maybe be exclusive in this respect because of our elaborate speech, but again, this is another unknown. However, eventually reflex breathing will always reclaim its command over breathing—as anyone who has performed a prolonged breath-hold will know.

Summary

So we have seen that at the heart of the control of breathing there is a pacemaker establishing a basic rhythm and depth of breathing, but this is influenced by numerous other factors from both the lung and higher brain. These influences adjust breathing via the brainstem to produce respiratory responses to the environment and changes in emotional state, and contribute to efficient and appropriate levels of ventilation.

Chemical Control of Breathing

It perhaps comes as no surprise that the major influence on the reflex drive to breathe comes from the homeostatic need to match ventilation with metabolic demand and maintain blood O_2, CO_2, and pH within narrow ranges. The chemoreflexes are therefore capable of sensing changes in arterial oxygen, carbon dioxide, and pH, modifying the activity of the brainstem respiratory centers and affecting an appropriate change in alveolar ventilation. These reflexes all act as classical negative feedback circuits and are capable of maintaining despite large changes in O_2 consumption and CO_2 production by metabolizing tissue.

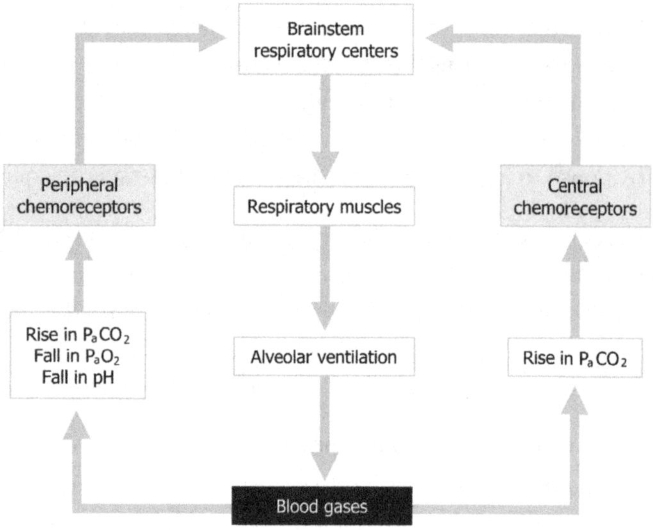

Figure 17.3: Chemoreflex circuit.

Before getting into the details of the chemoreceptors, let us take a quick overview of the basic circuitry of the chemoreflexes (figure 17.3). There are two sets of sensors in our circuit: the peripheral chemoreceptors that are in the vasculature, and the central chemoreceptors that are found on the surface of the brainstem. The central chemoreceptors are capable of detecting changes in arterial CO_2, while the peripheral chemoreceptors respond to changes in CO_2, O_2, and arterial pH.

Upon excitation by changes in blood gas values, the receptors fire back to the reflex's controller, the respiratory centers in the brainstem. This results in an increase in reflex ventilatory drive and a greater motor signal to the respiratory muscles. This produces an increase in alveolar ventilation that corrects the blood gas disturbances and stops the chemoreceptors from firing.

With that basic circuit in mind, let us now look more closely at the chemoreceptors and the ventilatory responses they can induce.

Central Chemoreceptors

We will start with the central chemoreceptors. The central chemoreceptors are comprised of chemosensitive neurons on the ventral surface of the medulla found close to the entry points of the glossopharyngeal and vagus nerves (coincidentally these are the nerves bringing in afferent information from the peripheral chemoreceptors and the pulmonary mechanoreceptors).

Although the central chemoreceptors do not respond to hypoxemia and only respond to rises in arterial CO_2, their activity accounts for about 80 percent of the hypercapnic ventilatory response. Given the critical importance of maintaining a normal P_aCO_2, these are considered the most important chemoreceptors for minute-by-minute regulation of ventilation. Ironically they do not respond to CO_2 directly, but rather to changes in pH of the cerebrospinal fluid (CSF).

This complication comes from the fact that the central chemoreceptors are not exposed to the blood, but rather are behind the blood brain barrier and bathed in CSF. Hydrogen ions and bicarbonate cannot pass through the blood brain barrier, but CO_2 can. Once through the blood brain barrier, CO_2 forms carbonic acid in the reaction that is very familiar to you. It is the hydrogen ion from the dissociated carbonic acid that stimulates the chemoreceptors. So the central chemoreceptors respond to a rise in arterial CO_2 via a change in CSF pH. Because there is little protein in the CSF, there is little buffering capability, and pH changes here tend to be greater than in the blood where plasma proteins are plentiful. This makes the central chemoreceptors quite sensitive and partly explains their substantial role in CO_2 control.

Prolonged exposure to high CO_2, such as in chronic lung disease, can lead to a rise in CSF bicarbonate. This bicarbonate buffers hydrogen ions and reduces the sensitivity of the central chemoreceptors. This partly explains why the hypercapnic ventilatory response diminishes over time in chronic lung patients, such as those with COPD.

Peripheral Chemoreceptors

The peripheral chemoreceptors are directly exposed to arterial blood and are capable of responding to changes in CO_2, O_2, and pH. There are two populations of chemoreceptive cells in the vasculature (see figure 17.4). One population is found in the aortic arch and is referred to as the aortic bodies. These are wired into the brainstem through afferent fibers that project to and join the vagus nerve. The other chemoreceptor is comprised of the carotid bodies, found in the bifurcation of the common carotid arteries. These connect to the brainstem through the carotid sinus and the glossopharyngeal nerves. The carotid bodies are by far the most important in humans, with the aortic bodies contributing very little to any ventilatory response.

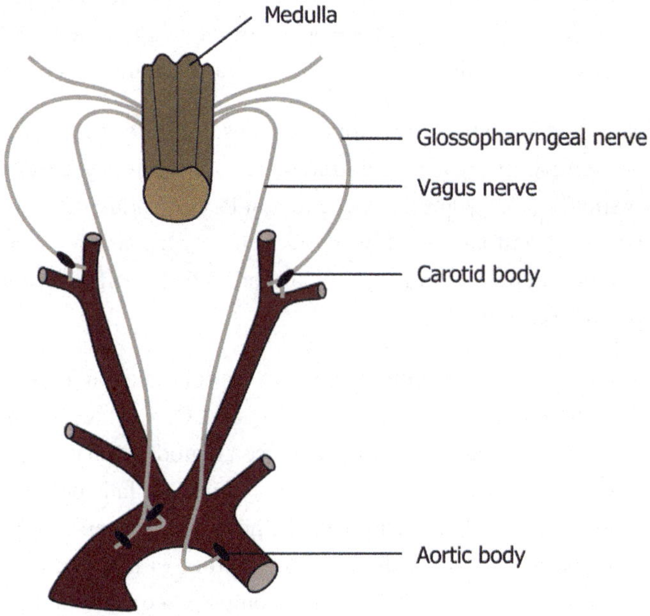

Figure 17.4: Peripheral chemoreceptors.

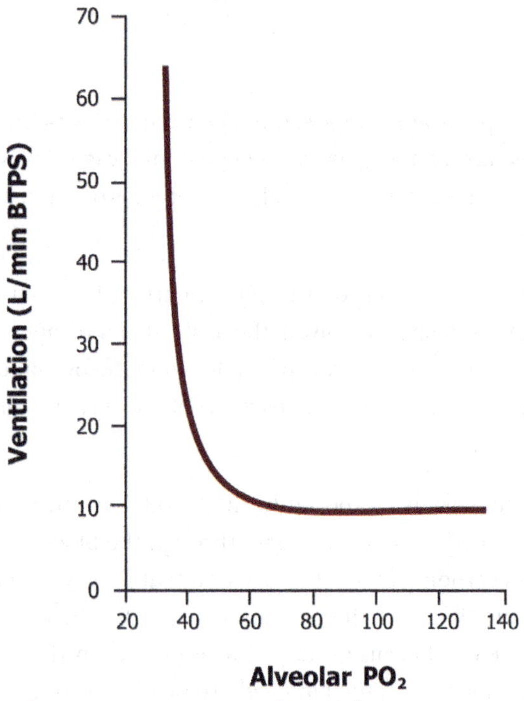

Figure 17.5: Hypoxic ventilatory response. BTPS: body temperature and pressure, saturated.

Although the carotid bodies play little role in reflex response to CO_2, their response to hypercapnia is more rapid than the central chemoreceptors and so they are capable of breath-by-breath regulation and responding to abrupt changes in arterial PCO_2. More importantly the peripheral chemoreceptors are entirely responsible for the response to hypoxia. The mechanism as to how these receptors work is unclear, but cells within the carotid bodies have very high metabolic rates and receive a proportionately high blood flow. It is likely that a decline in oxygen interrupts their metabolism and reduces their inhibitory interaction on neurotransmitter-filled neighboring cells, allowing excitation of the carotid sinus nerve. Their response to a decline in blood oxygen is far from linear. A decline in PO_2 below 100 mmHg causes little change in action potential firing, but the rate of firing rapidly increases at PO_2s below 50. This is reflected in the hypoxic ventilatory response illustrated in the graph in figure 17.5.

Figure 17.5 shows the hypoxic ventilatory response across a range of alveolar PO_2s at normal PCO_2. You can see that there is little increase in ventilation until alveolar PO_2 is below 55 mmHg, and then ventilation increases very rapidly. This is likely a reflection of the peripheral chemoreceptors, firing rate, which increases rapidly below PO_2 of 50 mmHg.

Because of this, the hypoxic ventilatory response normally plays little role in the control of breathing in humans. The hypoxic ventilatory response becomes more significant at altitude when inspired PO_2 is low, or more pertinently in lung disease, where alveolar ventilation or gas exchange is compromised.

The hypercapnic ventilatory response (figure 17.6) is much more influential on breathing in humans on a normal day-to-day basis. The response is very linear, with a rise in PCO_2 producing a proportionate rise in ventilation, driven of course primarily by the central chemoreceptors, but also contributed to by the afferent activity of the peripheral receptors.

The central and peripheral chemoreceptors keep arterial PCO_2 within very fine limits, primarily because of CO_2's effect on pH. Alveolar ventilation rapidly increases with even a moderate rise in arterial CO_2, but can completely stop (apnea) if arterial CO_2 falls below normal (~40 mmHg). The wakeful drive to breathe tends to keep CO_2 a little lower than the set-point of the chemoreceptors—a point illustrated during sleep, when the brainstem has complete control of breathing and P_aCO_2 is seen to rise a few mmHg.

The hypercapnic ventilatory response adapts to chronically elevated arterial CO_2, such as in severe lung disease. Here we not only see the CSF increase its buffering capacity with increased bicarbonate, but we also see the chemoreceptors change their set-point. It is not uncommon to see COPD patients with arterial PCO_2s above 60.

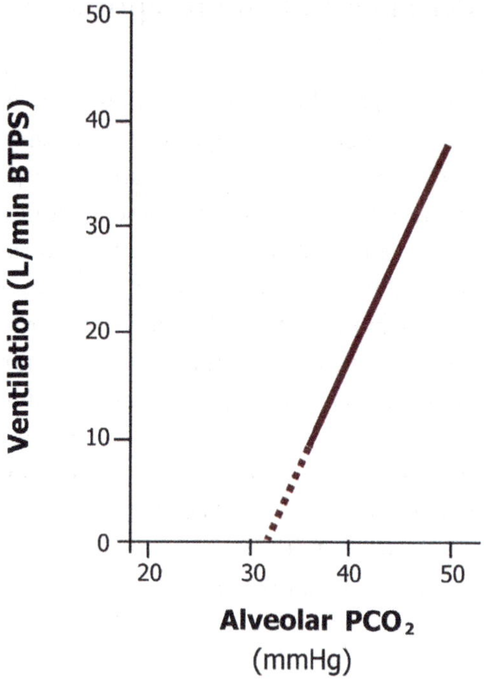

Figure 17.6: Hypercapnic ventilatory response.

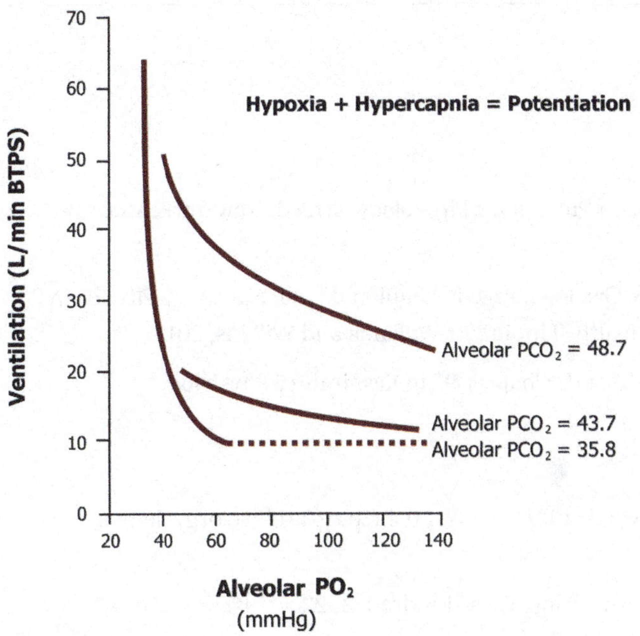

Figure 17.7: Hypoxic ventilatory responses with varying degrees of hypercapnia.

Finally, the hypoxic and hypercapnic ventilatory responses are not independent, and when they are both present at the same time a potentiation is seen (i.e., the response to hypoxic and hypercapnia is greater than the sum of the two individual responses).

The hypoxic ventilatory response we have just looked at was measured at an alveolar PCO_2 of 35.8 mmHg. If the same test is performed at higher PCO_2s (figure 17.7), then the hypoxic ventilatory response is much greater, as shown by these upwardly shifted lines when alveolar PCO_2 is set to 43.7 mmHg and 48.7 mmHg.

Likewise, the hypercapnic ventilatory response is exaggerated in the presence of hypoxia (see figure 17.8). The hypercapnic ventilatory response we have just looked at was measured at a "normal" alveolar PO_2 of 110 mmHg. If the hypercapnic response is measured in the presence of hypoxia, then the curve shifts upward, as shown by the upper lines when alveolar PO_2 is reduced to 47 mmHg and 37 mmHg. This potentiation likely comes from the peripheral chemoreceptors, whose firing rate is potentiated in the presence of both stimuli. Consequently, when a patient is both hypoxic and hypercapnic, then they are likely to have a very high drive to breathe, and when this occurs they are likely to feel very short of breath—the topic of the last chapter.

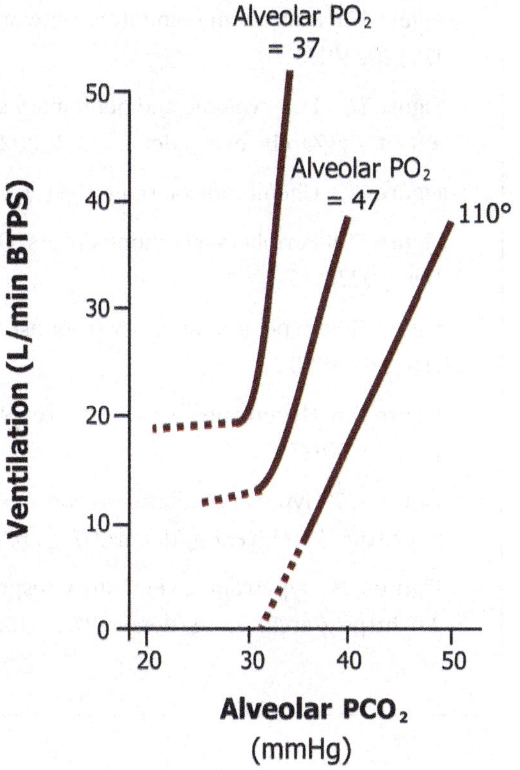

Figure 17.8: Hypercapnic ventilatory responses with varying degrees of hypoxia.

Summary

The chemoreflexes modulate breathing to maintain constant arterial blood gases and pH. These reflexes are initiated by central sensors that respond to hypoxia and peripheral sensors that respond to hypercapnia, hypoxia, and changes in arterial pH. Together these sensors can maintain arterial blood gases within narrow ranges despite large changes in oxygen consumption and CO_2 production associated with changes in metabolic rate.

References, Resources, and Further Reading

Text

Levitsky, Michael G. "Chapter 9: Control of Breathing." In *Pulmonary Physiology*, 9th ed. New York: McGraw Hill Education, 2018.

West, John B. "Chapter 8: Control of Ventilation—How Gas Exchange Is Regulated." In *Respiratory Physiology: The Essentials*, 9th ed. Philadelphia: Wolters Kluwer Health/Lippincott Williams and Wilkins, 2012.

Widdicombe, John G., and Andrew S. Davis. "Chapter 8" and "Chapter 9." In *Respiratory Physiology*. Baltimore: University Park Press, 1983.

Figures

Figure 17.1: Brain stem respiratory network. Grey, Kindred. 2022. CC BY 4.0. https://archive.org/details/17.1_20220125

Figure 17.2: Lung volume and pulmonary stretch receptor firing. Grey, Kindred. 2022. CC BY 4.0. https://archive.org/details/17.2_20220125

Figure 17.3: Chemoreflex circuit. Grey, Kindred. 2022. CC BY 4.0. https://archive.org/details/17.3_20220125

Figure 17.4: Peripheral chemoreceptors. Grey, Kindred. 2022. CC BY 4.0. https://archive.org/details/17.4_20220125

Figure 17.5: Hypoxic ventilatory response. Grey, Kindred. 2022. CC BY 4.0. https://archive.org/details/17.5_20220125

Figure 17.6: Hypercapnic ventilatory response. Grey, Kindred. 2022. CC BY 4.0. https://archive.org/details/17.6_20220125

Figure 17.7: Hypoxic ventilatory responses with varying degrees of hypercapnia. Grey, Kindred. 2022. CC BY 4.0. https://archive.org/details/17.7_20220125

Figure 17.8: Hypercapnic ventilatory responses with varying degrees of hypoxia. Grey, Kindred. 2022. CC BY 4.0. https://archive.org/details/17.8_20220125

18. Dyspnea

Learning objectives

- Describe the neural origins of the sensations of air hunger, effort to breathe, and chest tightness, and their prevalence in different disease states.

Occurrence and Forms of Dyspnea

Introduction

Dyspnea is the clinical term for "shortness of breath." However, the term "dyspnea" no longer describes one sensation but likely includes at least three distinctive sensations associated with breathing that have separate underlying neural mechanisms. This chapter will give you an overview of these sensations and the potential clinical importance of being able to distinguish them.

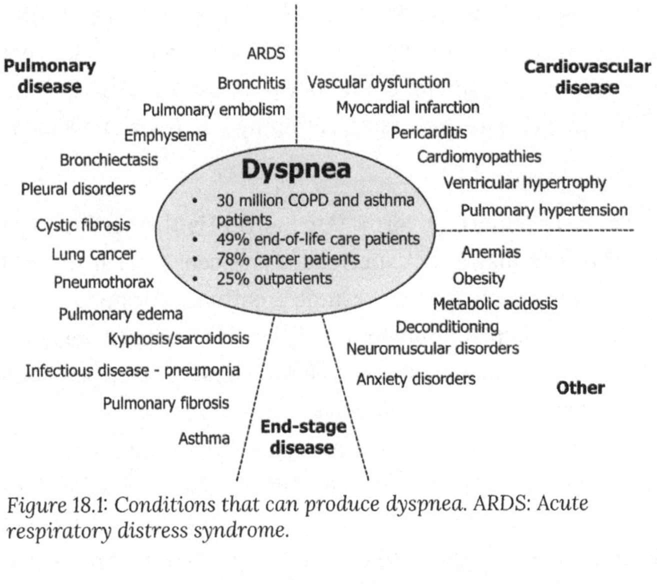

Figure 18.1: Conditions that can produce dyspnea. ARDS: Acute respiratory distress syndrome.

It might be worth putting dyspnea in a clinical context. Like pain, dyspnea can occur across a number of pathological conditions. It is the cardinal symptom of lung disease, but it is highly prevalent in heart diseases as well—in fact it is a more common sign of myocardial infarction in women than the classical symptom of chest pain that is more prevalent in men.

Dyspnea is also a strong predictor of mortality in most heart and lung diseases. As well as cardiopulmonary conditions, dyspnea is also prevalent in other conditions that affect breathing or metabolism, and (see figure 18.1) it is prevalent during end-stage disease where it is as common as pain and forms a significant problem for end-of-life care. Despite its prevalence there are few options for treating this symptom. Unlike pain, there are no specific drugs to reduce this sensation.

Forms of Dyspnea

So now let us look at the distinguishable sensations that the term dyspnea encompasses and begin to understand how they differ neurologically (see figure 18.2).

Effort to breathe: The first form of dyspnea is the sensation of work or effort to breathe. The healthy individual is usually unaware of the effort they are putting into breathing until breathing is significantly increased, such as during exercise when ventilation and work of breathing rises. The sensation of the work or effort to breathe is not particularly uncomfortable. If you jogged down the street now you might become more aware of the effort to breathe, but are not disturbed by it.

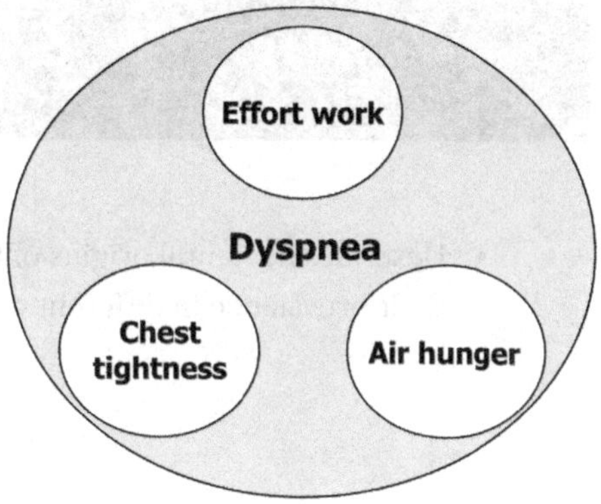

Figure 18.2: Types of dyspnea.

So where does this sensation come from?

An increase in motor drive is required to activate more tension or movement in any skeletal muscle, including the respiratory muscles. And like other skeletal muscles, such as limb muscles, we believe that the sensation of effort comes from a perception of that increased motor drive. Sensory information from the activated muscles, in our case the respiratory muscles, is thought to generate the sensation of work.

Getting laboratory subjects to report work and effort separately is very difficult, so for our purposes right now, we are grouping what might be two sensations together as one.

Chest tightness: The next form of dyspnea is primarily reported by asthmatic patients during bronchoconstriction. Similar to the sensation of work and effort, tightness was originally thought to arise from the increase in respiratory muscle activity associated with a rise in resistive work of breathing. But in 2002 we showed that "tightness" was unrelated to respiratory effort by removing respiratory muscle activity of bronchoconstricted asthmatics with mechanical ventilation. When we did this, "tightness" persisted, despite the respiratory muscles being inactive. So what does cause tightness? The next best, but so far unproven, alternative is that inflammation of the airways associated with an asthma attack leads to activation of airway irritant (or rapidly adapting) receptors, the afferent activity from which is perceived centrally as tightness.

Air hunger: Air hunger is arguably the most complex and clinically important form. "Air hunger" is the sensation of suffocation and can be described as a "desperate urge to breathe." You may have experienced this sensation at the end of a prolonged breath-hold, and it is the unpleasantness of air hunger that made you resume breathing. "Air hunger" is a warning signal that ventilation is insufficient and blood gases are becoming deranged; given the immediate importance of maintaining constant blood gases, air hunger is perhaps our most important homeostatic signal, and it has been referred to as the "suffocation alarm." The mechanisms underlying air hunger are still unclear, but again, they were once thought to involve the respiratory muscle motor and sensory signals and detection of a disparity between them—that is, the brain perceived that the respiratory muscles were not achieving the work they had been commanded to do. This hypothesis was developed in the sixties and still persists in texts today; however, it is wrong. In two separate labs, one at Harvard University and the other in Australia, pulmonary physiologists completely paralyzed each other to remove all motor activity; when they inhaled carbon dioxide, they still felt air hungry, suggesting the respiratory muscle signals were not essential to generate air hunger. So where does air hunger come from?

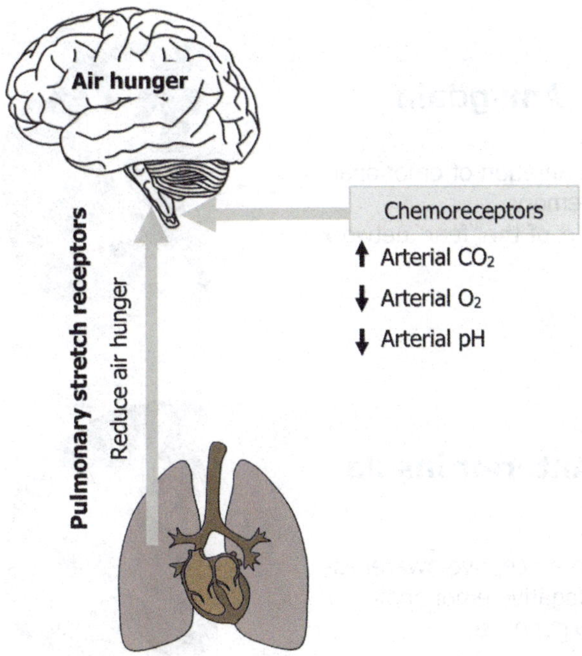

Figure 18.3: The proposed neural mechanism of air hunger.

We see air hunger arise when P_aCO_2 rises, when P_aO_2 falls, or when arterial pH decreases. These changes are detected by chemoreceptors that reflexly increase the drive to breathe from the brainstem. While we are not usually aware of our reflex breathing drive, we think that once this drive increases to a critical level, a signal is sent upward that is perceived as air hunger.

So any signals to the brainstem respiratory networks that increase the drive to breathe are likely to promote air hunger, and these influences may not all be chemical (see figure 18.3). For example, emotions such as anxiety increase the drive to breathe, and this is a pertinent point with clinical ramifications that we will return to.

Likewise, any influences that reduce the drive to breathe also have a tendency to reduce air hunger (see figure 18.3). Perhaps the most interesting example of this is the effect of pulmonary stretch receptor activity. Pulmonary stretch receptors are mechanoreceptors in the airways that respond to lung inflation. Although this pulmonary afferent activity is thought to have little effect on the control of breathing in man, it reduces the drive to breathe in other species as part of the Hering–Breuer reflex. What we see in humans is that lung inflation, and presumably an increase in pulmonary stretch receptor firing, profoundly reduces air hunger, even in the absence of any blood gas improvements.

This is easy to demonstrate to yourself by holding your breath; during the breath-hold CO_2 will gradually accumulate in your bloodstream and you will feel a gradually increasing urge to breathe that will become increasingly more uncomfortable to a point when it is intolerable and you must begin breathing again. That first big breath you take does not return your arterial CO_2 to normal, but despite this you get great relief from air hunger by taking it, probably because that big breath stretched the lung and caused a rapid increase of stretch receptor activity to the brainstem.

So air hunger is really affected by a balance of influences: those that increase the drive to breathe (such as hypercapnia and hypoxia) promote air hunger, while inhibitory influences on the drive to breathe tend to promote comfort (see figure 18.4).

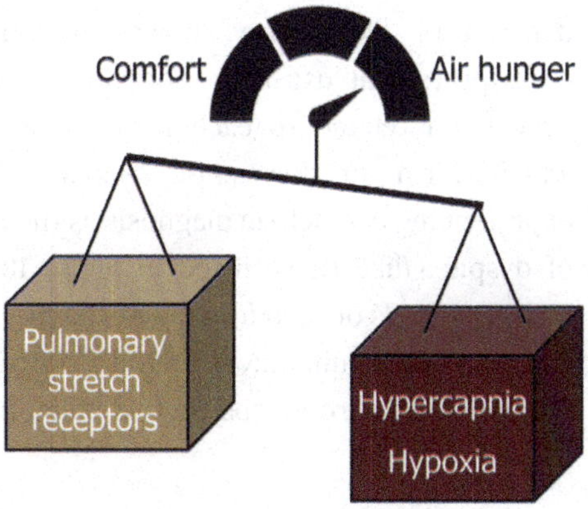

Figure 18.4: Balance of pulmonary stretch receptors and chemoreceptor firing.

Impact of Dyspnea

There are other elements that should be considered when dealing with the air-hungry patient. Probably because of its homeostatic importance, the sensation of air hunger is very effective at getting attention and producing fear and anxiety. Recent comparisons of attentive and emotional impacts suggest air hunger is perceived as much more threatening and worrisome than pain at equivalent intensities. (Ironically we routinely ask about patients' pain, but rarely about their air hunger.)

This emotional impact of air hunger is reflected in the regions of the brain that are consistently seen to be activated in recent functional brain imaging studies (see figure 18.5). The amygdala, anterior insula, and anterior cingulate are all persistently seen to activate during air hunger, and all are either associated with the brain's fear network or generation of emotional responses. The activation of the anterior insula is also interesting as this phylogenically old part of the cortex also responds to other homeostatic imbalances, such as thirst, hunger for food, and pain. Although air hunger itself is unpleasant, it is these emotional components that produce air hunger's profoundly negative effect on patients' quality of life and makes end-of-life distressing for both the patient and their loved ones. We will come back to the impact of emotional responses in a moment.

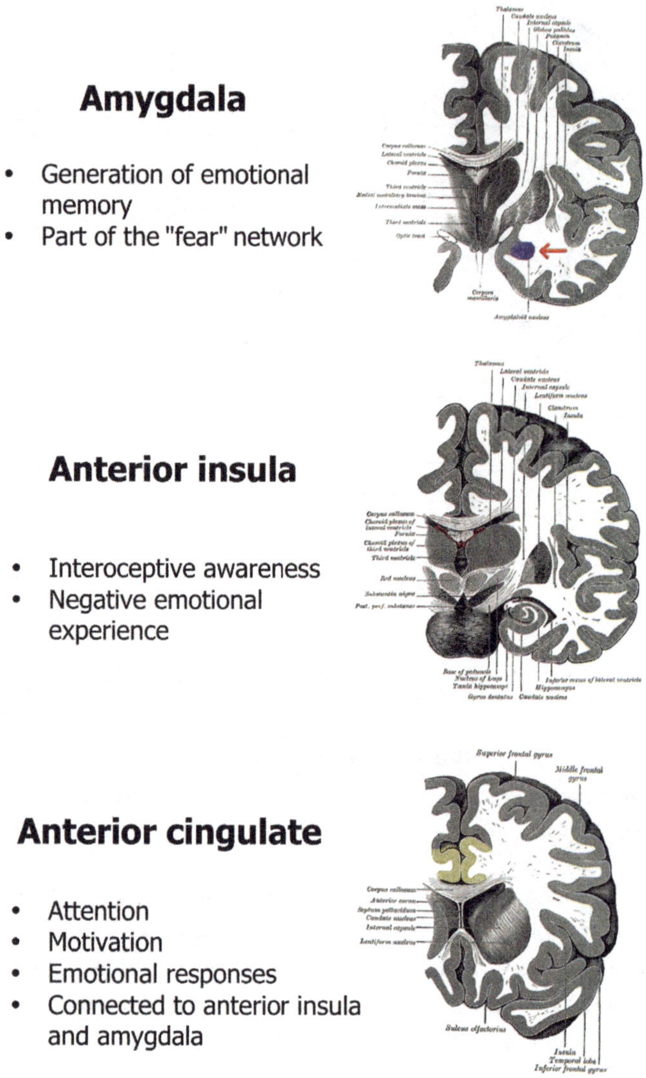

Figure 18.5: Central regions associated with air hunger.

So there we are—three different forms of dyspnea, with separate neural mechanisms. That said, it is unlikely that a patient will ever walk into your office and tell you they have "dyspnea," or pinpoint which form of dyspnea they have. But taking an interest in the subtleties of your patients' comments may not be a purely academic exercise either. More likely they are likely to use descriptors like those shown in table 18.1. These descriptors that use more common, everyday language have been related to each form of dyspnea. Knowing which form or forms of dyspnea the patient is experiencing can help in diagnosis as the different causes of dyspnea (like those listed in figure 18.1) can produce different levels of each form. For example, chest tightness is much more commonly reported by asthmatics, whereas patients with chronic obstructive pulmonary disease tend to use descriptors more related to effort to breathe and air hunger.

Form of dyspnea	Common descriptors
Air hunger	- I feel that I am suffocating - I feel out of breath - I cannot get enough air - I am gasping for air - My breath does not go in all the way - I feel a hunger for more air
Effort to breathe	- I feel that my breathing is rapid - I feel that I am breathing more - My breathing requires effort - My breathing is heavy - My breathing is shallow
Chest tightness	- My chest feels tight - My chest is constricted

Table 18.1: Patient descriptors for the three different forms of dyspnea.

While the different forms of dyspnea have been investigated, described, and now explored as their potential as diagnostic tools, the emotional impact of dyspnea is only now receiving more attention. The most immediate complication caused by the emotional component is the potential for a positive feedback loop to form between air hunger and the anxiety it generates. The anxiety that air hunger produces results in an increased drive to breathe; in turn this increased drive to breathe causes the air hunger to increase, which leads to more anxiety and so on (figure 18.6).

Behavioral effects of dyspnea: This cycle can be entered into by different types of patients; those with cardiopulmonary disease enter the cycle at the point of the air hunger, whereas patients with anxiety disorders can enter the cycle at this point and can experience significant air hunger even with apparently perfectly normal lung and heart function. On a more long-term basis the quality of life of air-hungry patients can be diminished by another positive feedback scenario that can produce "respiratory cripples" of cardiopulmonary patients. The air hunger produced by the underlying disease worsens during exertion, so makes exercising uncomfortable. This frequently results in patients avoiding exercise, perhaps starting with taking an elevator instead of the stairs, or driving to the grocery store when previously they might have walked.

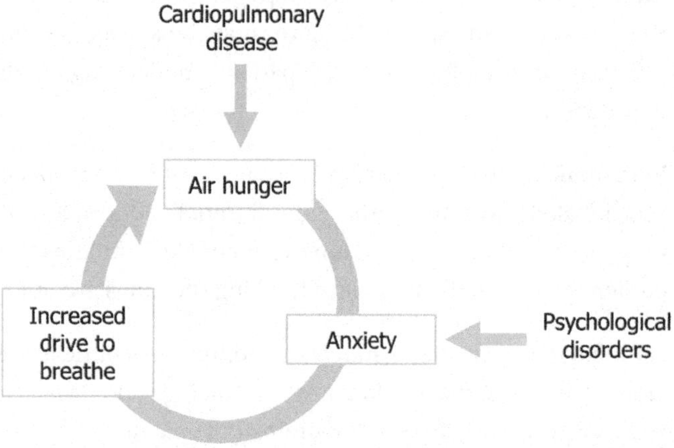

Figure 18.6: The cycle of anxiety causing an increase in the drive to breathe and air hunger, which in turn causes more anxiety. Psychological disorders can produce air hunger if they involve anxiety.

This reduction in exercise leads to cardiac deconditioning, which in turn makes the air hunger worse and leads to further avoidance of exercise. Along with the progression of the disease, this cycle may leave the patient out-of-breath while simply sitting in a chair.

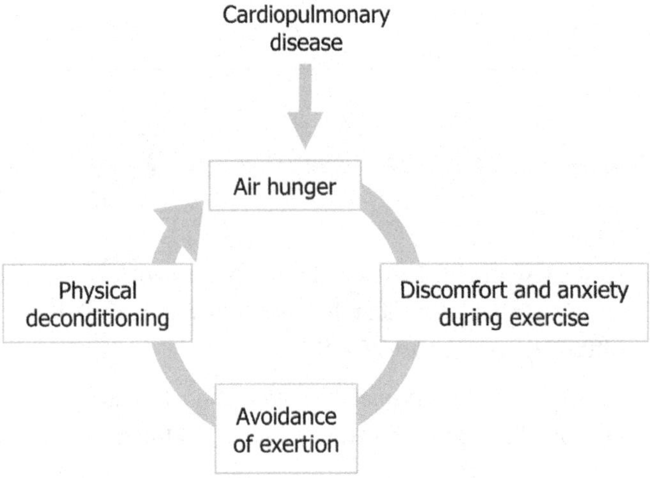

Figure 18.7: The cycle of worsening air hunger leading to exercise avoidance and physical deconditioning, which in turn worsens the air hunger during exertion.

The patient's quality of life becomes severely diminished as their life is ruled by dyspnea that prevents them from leaving the house, interacting with children or grandchildren, and performing simple activities that used to bring enjoyment, such as gardening, wood-working, walking, and more. This reduced quality of life can potentially lead to depression, and the emotional response to dyspnea may be exacerbated.

So what can be done to relieve the patient's air hunger and the associated anxiety? Well, despite its prevalence, the treatment of dyspnea is decades behind the treatment of pain. For too long the approach to treating dyspnea has been to treat the underlying disease with the expectation that the dyspnea will go away. This is true and a perfect course of action for many conditions, but for many diseases that produce dyspnea we have ineffective cures, such as emphysema, lung cancer, and pulmonary fibrosis. How do we make the 49 percent of terminally ill patients who suffer with dyspnea at the end of life more comfortable?

Opioids: A common practice is to use opioids, but the mechanism of how they might work and indeed their overall efficacy has been disputed. There are a number of routes for how morphine may act, if it indeed does so. Opioids may have a direct inhibitory effect on the central networks that generate air hunger, or at higher dose concentrations they may reduce air hunger indirectly by causing respiratory depression—that is, they tackle air hunger at what we think to be its source. Alternatively, opioids may reduce the affective or emotional component of dyspnea (i.e., the patient may perceive air hunger, but simply is not as bothered by it). Recent work from Harvard University suggests that morphine has a direct effect on both the sensory and affective components of air hunger independent of its effect on ventilatory drive.

Anxiolytics: As the emotional component of air hunger is so strong, the fear and anxiety produced can be treated in the absence of any specific drug to treat the air hunger itself. Use of anxiolytics drugs has also produced mixed results that may be complicated by the patient's underlying condition, and whether the type of anxiolytic causes ventilatory depression.

Furosemide: Although there is currently no drug that specifically tackles air hunger, there is a growing body of evidence that inhaled furosemide (the loop diuretic) reduces air hunger by sensitizing pulmonary stretch receptors, meaning they fire more for any given lung volume. This amplifies the stretch receptors' inhibitory effect on air hunger described earlier, by fooling the brain into thinking the lungs are at a greater volume than they really are.

Nonpharmaceutical alternatives: A nonpharmaceutical alternative is to simply cool the patient's face with a fan or wet cloth. This facial cooling initiates the "diving reflex" via the trigeminal nerve. One component of the diving reflex is to reduce ventilatory drive at the brainstem—an ideal response if one is heading underwater.

This inhibition of ventilatory drive is likely responsible for the moderate reduction in air hunger seen with facial cooling.

Rehabilitation and desensitization: While dyspnea can be addressed by other methods than those briefly described here, few have been shown to work consistently or effectively. On a more long-term basis, breathing training and pulmonary rehabilitation appear to help patients overcome exacerbations of their disease or even reduce chronic air hunger, but both require patient cooperation and compliance and may have limited effect in severe disease. What can be taken from the literature is that the treatment of dyspnea is in desperate need of more attention. For a symptom that is so common and has such an impact on patients, dyspnea is a clinical issue that is woefully underaddressed.

References, Resources, and Further Reading

Text

American Thoracic Society Committee on Dyspnea. "An Official American Thoracic Society Statement: Update on the Mechanisms, Assessment, and Management of Dyspnea." American Journal of Respiratory and Critical Care Medicine 185, no. 4: 435–52. https://doi.org/10.1164/rccm.201111-2042ST.

Banzett, Robert B., Robert W. Lansing, and Andrew P. Binks. "Air Hunger: A Primal Sensation and a Primary Element of Dyspnea." Comprehensive Physiology 11, no. 2 (April 2021): 1449–83. https://doi.org/10.1002/cphy.c200001.

Figures

Figure 18.1: Conditions that can produce dyspnea. Grey, Kindred. 2022. CC BY 4.0. https://archive.org/details/18.1_20220125

Figure 18.2: Types of dyspnea. Grey, Kindred. 2022. CC BY 4.0. https://archive.org/details/18.2_20220125

Figure 18.3: The proposed neural mechanism of air hunger. Grey, Kindred. 2022. CC BY 4.0. Added Brain by Clockwise from Noun Project. CC BY 3.0. https://archive.org/details/18.3_20220125

Figure 18.4: Balance of pulmonary stretch receptor and chemoreceptor firing. Grey, Kindred. 2022. CC BY 4.0. Added credit score by akash k from Noun Project. CC BY 3.0. https://archive.org/details/18.4_20220125

Figure 18.5: Central regions associated with air hunger. Grey, Kindred. 2022. CC BY 4.0. Added Gray 718-amygdala by Henry Vandyke Carter from WikimediaCommons. Public domain. Added Gray717 by Henry Vandyke Carter from WikimediaCommons. Public domain. Added Gray743 cingulate gyrus by Henry Vandyke Carter (colored by was_a_bee) from WikimediaCommons. Public domain. https://archive.org/details/

17.5-needs-numbering/mode/1up
Figure 18.6: The cycle of anxiety causing an increase in the drive to breathe and air hunger. Grey, Kindred. 2022. CC BY 4.0. https://archive.org/details/18.6_20220125/mode/1up

Figure 18.7: The cycle of worsening air hunger leading to exercise avoidance and physical deconditioning. Grey, Kindred. 2022. CC BY 4.0. https://archive.org/details/18.7_20220125/mode/1up

Made in the USA
Monee, IL
02 November 2026

67377398R00063